Contents

Heart Disease: Why Should You Care?

If you're like many people, you may think of heart disease as a problem that happens to *other* folks. "I feel fine," you may think, "so I have nothing to worry about." If you're a woman, you may also believe that being female protects you from heart disease. If you're a man, you may think you're not old enough to have a serious heart condition.

Wrong on all counts. In the United States, heart disease is the #1 killer of both women and men. It affects many people at midlife, as well as in old age. It also can happen to those who "feel fine." Consider these facts:

- Each year, 500,000 Americans die of heart disease, and approximately half of them are women.
- As early as age 45, a man's risk of heart disease begins to rise significantly. For a woman, risk starts to increase at age 55.
- Fifty percent of men and 64 percent of women who die suddenly of heart disease have no previous symptoms of the disease.

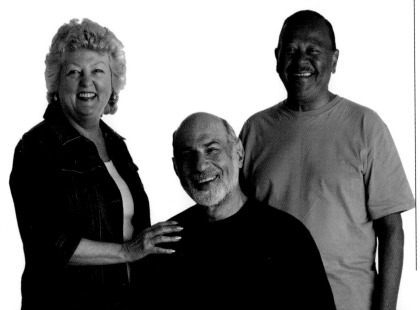

These facts may seem frightening, but they need not be. The good news is that you have a lot of power to protect and improve your heart health. This guidebook will help you find out your own risk of heart disease and take steps to prevent it.

"But," you may still be thinking, "I take pretty good care of myself. I'm unlikely to get heart disease." Yet a recent national survey shows that only 3 percent of U.S. adults practice all of the "Big Four" habits that help to prevent heart disease: eating a healthy diet, getting regular physical activity, maintaining a healthy weight, and avoiding smoking. Many young people are also vulnerable. A recent study showed that about two-thirds of teenagers already have at least one risk factor for heart disease.

Every risk factor counts. Research shows that each individual risk factor greatly increases the chances of developing heart disease. Moreover, the worse a particular risk factor is, the more likely you are to develop heart disease. For example, if you have high blood pressure, the higher it is, the greater your chances of developing heart disease, including its many serious consequences. A damaged heart can damage your life by interfering with enjoyable activities, preventing you from holding a job, and even keeping you from doing simple things, such as taking a walk or climbing steps.

What can you do to reduce your personal risk of heart disease? First, you can learn about your own risk factors. Second, you can begin to make healthful changes in your diet, physical activity, and other daily habits. Whatever your age or current state of health, it's never too late to take steps to protect your heart. It's also never too early. The sooner you act, the better. So use this guidebook to find out more about the state of your heart, and to learn about heart healthy living. Talk with your doctor to get more information. Start taking action to improve your heart health today.

What You Need To Know About Heart Disease

What Is Heart Disease?

Coronary heart disease—often simply called heart disease—occurs when the arteries that supply blood to the heart muscle become hardened and narrowed due to a buildup of plaque on the arteries' inner walls. Plaque is the accumulation of fat, cholesterol, and other substances. As plaque continues to build up in the arteries, blood flow to the heart is reduced.

Heart disease can lead to a heart attack. A heart attack happens when an artery becomes totally blocked with plaque, preventing vital oxygen and nutrients from getting to the heart. A heart attack can cause permanent damage to the heart muscle.

Heart disease is one of several cardiovascular diseases, which are disorders of the heart and blood vessel system. Other cardiovascular diseases include stroke, high blood pressure, and rheumatic heart disease.

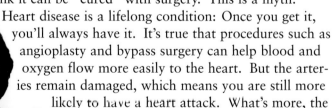

Some people aren't too concerned about heart disease because they think it can be "cured" with surgery. This is a myth. Heart disease is a lifelong condition: Once you get it, you'll always have it. It's true that procedures such as angioplasty and bypass surgery can help blood and oxygen flow more easily to the heart. But the arteries remain damaged, which means you are still more likely to have a heart attack. What's more, the condition of your blood vessels will steadily worsen unless you make changes in your daily habits and control your risk factors. Many people die of complications from heart disease, or become permanently disabled. That's why it is so vital to take action to prevent this disease.

Who Is at Risk?

Risk factors are conditions or habits that make a person more likely to develop a disease. They can also increase the chances that an existing disease will get worse. Important risk factors for heart disease that you can do something about are cigarette smoking, high blood pressure, high blood cholesterol, overweight, physical inactivity, and diabetes. Recent research shows that more than 95 percent of those who die from heart disease have at least one of these major risk factors.

Certain risk factors, such as getting older, can't be changed. After menopause, women are more likely to develop heart disease. For both women and men, middle age is a time of increasing risk because people are more likely to develop heart disease risk factors during this stage of life.

Family history of early heart disease is another risk factor that can't be changed. If your father or brother had a heart attack before age 55, or if your mother or sister had one before age 65, you are more likely to get heart disease.

While certain risk factors cannot be changed, it is important to realize that you *do* have control over many others. Regardless of your age or family history, you can take important steps to lower your risk of heart disease.

How Risk Works

It may be tempting to believe that doing just one healthy thing will take care of your heart disease risk. For example, you may hope that if you walk or swim regularly, you can still eat a lot of fatty foods and stay fairly healthy. Not true. To protect your heart, it is vital to make changes that address each and every risk factor you have. You can make the changes gradually, one at a time. But making them is very important.

While each risk factor increases your risk of heart disease, having more than one risk factor is especially serious. That's because risk factors tend to "gang up" and worsen each other's effects. For example, if you have high blood cholesterol and you smoke, your heart disease risk increases enormously. The message is clear: You need to take heart disease risk seriously, and the best time to reduce that risk is now.

What's Your Risk?

The first step toward heart health is becoming aware of your own personal risk for heart disease. Some risks, such as smoking cigarettes or being overweight, are obvious: All of us know whether we smoke or whether we need to lose a few pounds. But other risk factors, such as high blood pressure or high blood cholesterol, have few visible signs or symptoms. So you'll need to gather some information to create your own personal "heart profile."

How To Talk With Your Doctor

The first step in finding out your risk is to make an appointment with your doctor for a thorough checkup. Your physician can be an important partner in helping you set and reach goals for heart health. But don't wait for your doctor to mention heart disease or its risk factors. Many physicians don't routinely bring up the topic, especially with their female patients. New research shows that women are less likely than men to receive heart healthy recommendations from their doctors. Here's how to speak up and establish good, clear communication between you and your doctor.

Ask for what you need. Tell your doctor that you want to keep your heart healthy and would like help in achieving that goal. Ask questions about your chances of developing heart disease and ways to lower your risk. (See "Questions To Ask Your Doctor" on the next page.) Also ask for tests that will determine your personal risk factors. (See "What's Your Number?" on page 8.)

Be open. When your doctor asks you questions, answer them as honestly and fully as you can. While certain topics may seem quite personal,

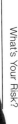

discussing them openly can help your doctor find out your chances of developing heart disease. It can also help your doctor work more effectively with you to reduce your risk.

Keep it simple. If you don't understand something your doctor says, ask for an explanation in plain language. Be especially sure you understand why and how to take any medication you're given. If you are worried about understanding what the doctor says, or if you have trouble hearing, bring a friend or relative with you to your appointment. You may want to ask that person to write down the doctor's instructions for you.

Questions To Ask Your Doctor

Getting answers to these questions will give you important information about your heart health and what you can do to improve it. You may want to bring this list to your doctor's office.

1. What is my risk for heart disease?
2. What is my blood pressure? What does it mean for me, and what do I need to do about it?
3. What are my cholesterol numbers? (These include total cholesterol, low-density lipoprotein (LDL) "bad" cholesterol, high-density lipoprotein (HDL) "good" cholesterol, and triglycerides.) What do they mean for me, and what do I need to do about them?
4. What are my body mass index (BMI) and waist measurement? Do they indicate that I need to lose weight for my health?
5. What is my blood sugar level? Does it mean I'm at risk for diabetes?
6. What other screening tests for heart disease do I need? How often should I return for checkups for my heart health?
7. For smokers: What can you do to help me quit smoking?
8. How much physical activity do I need to help protect my heart? What kinds of activities are helpful?
9. What is a heart healthy eating plan for me? Should I see a registered dietitian or qualified nutritionist to learn more about healthy eating?
10. How can I tell if I'm having a heart attack?

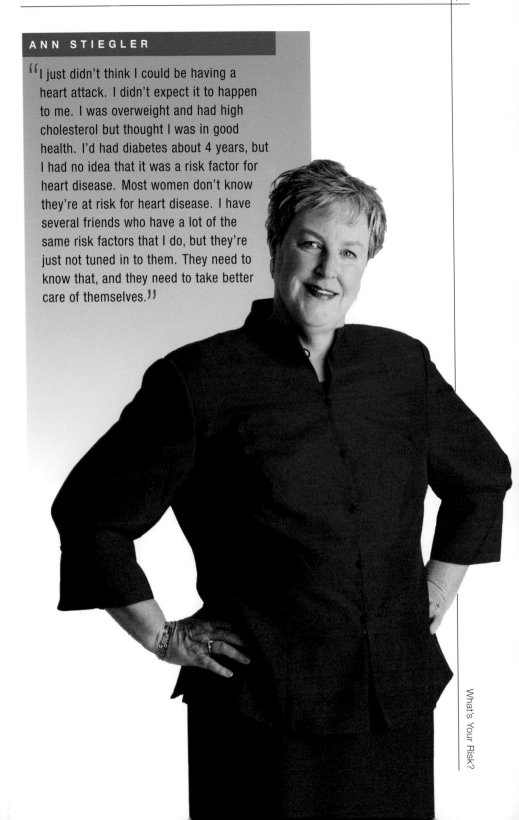

ANN STIEGLER

"I just didn't think I could be having a heart attack. I didn't expect it to happen to me. I was overweight and had high cholesterol but thought I was in good health. I'd had diabetes about 4 years, but I had no idea that it was a risk factor for heart disease. Most women don't know they're at risk for heart disease. I have several friends who have a lot of the same risk factors that I do, but they're just not tuned in to them. They need to know that, and they need to take better care of themselves."

What's Your Number?
Tests That Can Help Protect Your Health

Ask your doctor to give you these tests. Each one will give you valuable information about your heart disease risk.

Lipoprotein Profile

What: A blood test that measures total cholesterol, LDL "bad" cholesterol, HDL "good" cholesterol, and triglycerides (another form of fat in the blood). The test is given after a 9- to 12-hour fast.

Why: To find out if you have any of the following: high blood cholesterol (high total and LDL cholesterol), low HDL cholesterol, or high triglyceride levels. All affect your risk for heart disease.

When: All healthy adults should have a lipoprotein profile done at least once every 5 years. Depending on the results, your doctor may want to repeat the test more frequently.

Blood Pressure

What: A simple, painless test using an inflatable arm cuff.

Why: To find out if you have high blood pressure (also called hypertension) or prehypertension. Both are risk factors for heart disease.

When: At least every 2 years, or more often if you have high blood pressure or prehypertension.

Fasting Plasma Glucose

What: The preferred test for diagnosing diabetes. After you have fasted overnight, you will be given a blood test the following morning.

Why: To find out if you have diabetes or are likely to develop the disease. Fasting plasma glucose levels of 126 mg/dL or higher in two tests on different days mean that you have diabetes. Levels between 100 and 125 mg/dL mean that you have an increased risk of developing diabetes and may have prediabetes. Diabetes is an important risk factor for heart disease and other medical disorders.

When: At least every 3 years, beginning at age 45. If you have risk factors for diabetes, you should be tested at a younger age and more often.

Body Mass Index (BMI) and Waist Circumference

What: BMI is a measure of your weight in relation to your height. Waist circumference is a measure of the fat around your middle.

Why: To find out if your body type raises your risk of heart disease. A BMI of 25 or higher means you are overweight. A BMI of 30 or higher means you are obese. Both overweight and obesity are risk factors for heart disease. For women, a waist measurement of more than 35 inches increases the risk of heart disease and other serious health conditions. For men, a waist measurement of more than 40 inches increases risk.

When: Every 2 years, or more often if your doctor recommends it.

There are also several tests that can determine whether you already have heart disease. Ask your doctor whether you need a stress test, an electrocardiogram (ECG or EKG), or another diagnostic test.

What's Your Number?

Rating
Your Risk

Here is a quick quiz to find out if you have an increased risk for a heart attack. If you don't know some of the answers, ask your health care provider.

- Do you smoke?
- Is your blood pressure 140/90 mmHg or higher; OR, have you been told by your doctor that your blood pressure is too high?
- Has your doctor told you that your LDL "bad" cholesterol is too high; that your total cholesterol level is 200 mg/dL or higher; OR, that your HDL "good" cholesterol is less than 40 mg/dL?
- Has your father or brother had a heart attack before age 55; OR, has your mother or sister had one before age 65?
- Do you have diabetes OR a fasting blood sugar of 126 mg/dL or higher; OR, do you need medicine to control your blood sugar?
- For women: Are you over 55 years old?
- For men: Are you over 45 years old?
- Do you have a Body Mass Index score of 25 or more? (To find out, see page 27.)
- Do you get less than a total of 30 minutes of physical activity on most days?
- Has a doctor told you that you have angina (chest pains); OR, have you had a heart attack?

If you answered "yes" to any of these questions, you have a higher risk of having a heart attack. Read on to learn what you can do to lower your risk.

Rating Your Risk

Major Risk Factors

A strong partnership with your doctor is a vital first step in protecting your heart health. But to make a lasting difference, you'll also need to learn more about heart disease and the kinds of habits and conditions that can increase your risk. It's your heart, and you're in charge. What follows is a guide to the most important risk factors for heart disease and how each of them affects your health.

Smoking

Smoking is "the leading cause of preventable death and disease in the United States," according to the Centers for Disease Control and Prevention (CDC). People who smoke are up to six times more likely to suffer a heart attack than nonsmokers, and the risk increases with the number of cigarettes smoked each day. Smoking can also shorten a healthy life, because smokers are likely to suffer a heart attack or other major heart problem at least 10 years sooner than nonsmokers.

But heart disease is far from the only health risk faced by smokers. Smoking also raises the risk of stroke and greatly increases the chances of developing lung cancer. Smoking is also linked with many other types of cancer, including cancers of the mouth, urinary tract, kidney, and cervix. Smoking also causes most cases of chronic obstructive lung disease, which includes bronchitis and emphysema. If you live or work with others, your secondhand smoke can cause numerous health problems in those individuals. A recent study shows a 60-percent increased risk of heart disease for nonsmokers who are regularly exposed to secondhand smoke.

Currently, 25 percent of American men and 20 percent of American women are smokers. Even more disturbing, 26 percent of high school seniors smoke. In young people, smoking can interfere with lung growth and cause more frequent and severe respiratory illnesses, in addition to heart disease and cancer risks. The younger people start smoking cigarettes, the more likely they are to become strongly addicted to nicotine.

There is simply no safe way to smoke. Low-tar and low-nicotine cigarettes do not lessen the risks of heart disease or other smoking-related diseases. The only safe and healthful course is not to smoke at all. (For tips on quitting, see "You *Can* Stop Smoking" on page 76.)

High Blood Pressure

High blood pressure, also known as hypertension, is another major risk factor for heart disease, as well as for kidney disease and congestive heart failure. High blood pressure is also the most important risk factor for stroke. Even slightly high blood pressure levels increase your risk for these conditions.

New research shows that at least 65 million adults in the United States have high blood pressure—a 30-percent increase over the last several years. Equally worrisome, blood pressure levels have increased substantially for American children and teens, which increases their risk of developing hypertension in adulthood.

Major contributors to high blood pressure are a family history of the disease, overweight, and dietary salt. Older individuals are at higher risk than younger people. Among older individuals, women are more likely than men to develop high blood pressure. African Americans are more likely to develop high blood pressure, and at earlier ages, than Whites. But nearly all of us are at risk, especially as we grow older. Middle-aged Americans who don't currently have high blood pressure have a 90-percent chance of eventually developing the disease.

High blood pressure is often called the silent killer because it usually doesn't cause symptoms. As a result, many people pay little attention to their blood pressure until they become seriously ill. According to a national survey, two-thirds of people with high blood pressure do not have it under control. The good news is that you can take action to control or prevent high blood pressure, and thereby avoid many life-threatening disorders. A new blood pressure category, called prehypertension, has been created to alert people to their increased risk of developing high blood pressure so that they can take steps to prevent the disease.

What Is Blood Pressure?

Blood pressure is the amount of force exerted by the blood against the walls of the arteries. Everyone has to have some blood pressure, so that blood can get to all of the body's organs. Usually, blood pressure is expressed as two numbers, such as 120/80, and is measured in millimeters of mercury (mmHg). The first number is the systolic blood pressure, the amount of force used when the heart beats. The second number, or diastolic blood pressure, is the pressure that exists in the arteries between heartbeats.

Because blood pressure changes often, your health care provider should check it on several different days before deciding whether it is too high. Blood pressure is considered "high" when it stays above prehypertensive levels over a period of time. (See accompanying box.)

Your Blood Pressure:
Crunching the Numbers

Your blood pressure category is determined by the higher number of *either* your systolic or your diastolic measurement. For example, if your systolic number is 115 but your diastolic number is 85, your category is prehypertension.

	Systolic		Diastolic
Normal blood pressure	Less than 120 mmHg	and	Less than 80 mmHg
Prehypertension	120–139 mmHg	or	80–89 mmHg
High blood pressure	140 mmHg or higher	or	90 mmHg or higher

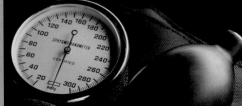

Blood Pressure

Understanding Risk

It's important to understand what each of these categories means. High blood pressure, of course, increases heart disease risk more than any other category. But many people don't realize that the second category—prehypertension—also increases your risk of heart attack, stroke, and heart failure. To the extent possible, everyone should aim for normal blood pressure levels.

Be aware, too, that a high systolic blood pressure level (first number) is dangerous. If your systolic blood pressure is 140 mmHg or higher, you are more likely to develop cardiovascular and kidney diseases even if your diastolic blood pressure (second number) is in the normal range. After age 50, people are more likely to develop high systolic blood pressure. High systolic blood pressure is high blood pressure. If you have this condition, you will need to take steps to control it. High blood pressure can be controlled in two ways: by changing your lifestyle and by taking medication.

Changing Your Lifestyle

If your blood pressure is not too high, you may be able to control it entirely by losing weight if you are overweight, getting regular physical activity, cutting down on alcohol, and changing your eating habits. A special eating plan called DASH can help you lower your blood pressure. DASH stands for "Dietary Approaches to Stop Hypertension." The DASH eating plan emphasizes fruits, vegetables, whole-grain foods, and low-fat or fat-free milk and milk products. It is rich in magnesium, potassium, and calcium, as well as protein and fiber. It is low in saturated and total fat and cholesterol, and limits red meat, sweets, and beverages with added sugars.

If you follow the DASH eating plan and also consume less sodium, you are likely to reduce your blood pressure even more. Sodium is a substance that affects blood pressure. It is the main ingredient in salt and is found in many processed foods, such as soups, convenience meals, some breads and cereals, and salted snacks.

For more on the DASH eating plan and other changes you can make to lower and prevent high blood pressure, see the "Taking Charge" section of this guidebook (pages 45–82.)

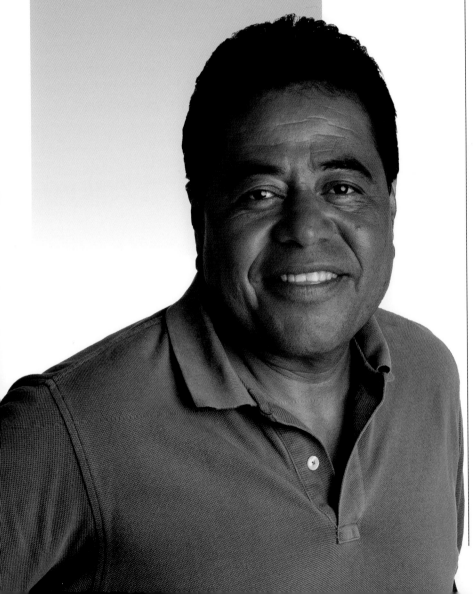

JOSE HENRIQUEZ

" The doctor sent me to a dietitian. She is the one who taught me the things that I had to do in order to eat right. It was hard at the beginning because once you have bad habits, they are hard to break. But, once I realized it was for my own good and no one was going to take care of me except me, I decided to start eating better. "

Taking Medication

If your blood pressure remains high even after you make lifestyle changes, your doctor will probably prescribe medicine. Lifestyle changes will help the medicine work more effectively. In fact, if you are successful with the changes you make in your daily habits, you may be able to gradually reduce how much medication you take.

Taking medicine to lower blood pressure can reduce your risk of stroke, heart attack, congestive heart failure, and kidney disease. If you take a drug and notice any uncomfortable side effects, ask your doctor about changing the dosage or switching to another type of medicine.

A recent study found that diuretics (water pills) work better than newer drugs to treat hypertension and prevent some forms of heart disease. If you're starting treatment for high blood pressure, try a diuretic first. If you need more than one drug, ask your doctor about making one of them a diuretic. If you're already taking

Preventing
Congestive Heart Failure

High blood pressure is the #1 risk factor for congestive heart failure. Heart failure is a life-threatening condition in which the heart cannot pump enough blood to supply the body's needs. Congestive heart failure occurs when excess fluid starts to leak into the lungs, causing tiredness, weakness, and breathing difficulties.

To prevent congestive heart failure and stroke as well, you must control your high blood pressure to below 140/90 mmHg. If your blood pressure is higher than that, talk with your doctor about starting or adjusting medication, as well as making lifestyle changes.

To avoid congestive heart failure, controlling your weight is also very important. Being even moderately overweight increases your risk of developing heart failure.

Congestive Heart Failure

medicine for high blood pressure, ask about switching to or adding a diuretic. Diuretics work for most people, but if you need a different drug, others are very effective. To make the best choice, talk with your doctor.

A reminder: It is important to take blood pressure medication exactly as your doctor has prescribed it. Before you leave your doctor's office, make sure you understand the amount of medicine you are supposed to take each day, and the specific times of day you should take it.

High Blood Cholesterol

High blood cholesterol is another major risk factor for heart disease that you can do something about. The higher your blood cholesterol level, the greater your risk for developing heart disease or having a heart attack. To prevent these disorders, you should make a serious effort to keep your cholesterol at healthy levels. Cholesterol lowering is important for everyone—women and men; younger, middle-aged, and older adults; and people with and without heart disease.

Cholesterol and Your Heart

The body needs cholesterol to function normally. However, your body makes all the cholesterol it needs. Over a period of years, extra cholesterol and fat circulating in the blood build up in the walls of the arteries that supply blood to the heart. This buildup, called plaque, makes the arteries narrower and narrower. As a result, less blood gets to the heart. Blood carries oxygen to the heart; if enough oxygen-rich blood cannot reach your heart, you may suffer chest pain. If the blood supply to a portion of the heart is completely cut off, the result is a heart attack.

Cholesterol travels in the blood in packages called lipoproteins. LDL carries most of the cholesterol in the blood. Cholesterol packaged in LDL is often called bad cholesterol, because too high a level of LDL in your blood can lead to cholesterol buildup and blockage in your arteries.

Another type of cholesterol is HDL, also called good cholesterol. That's because HDL helps remove cholesterol from the body, preventing it from building up in your arteries.

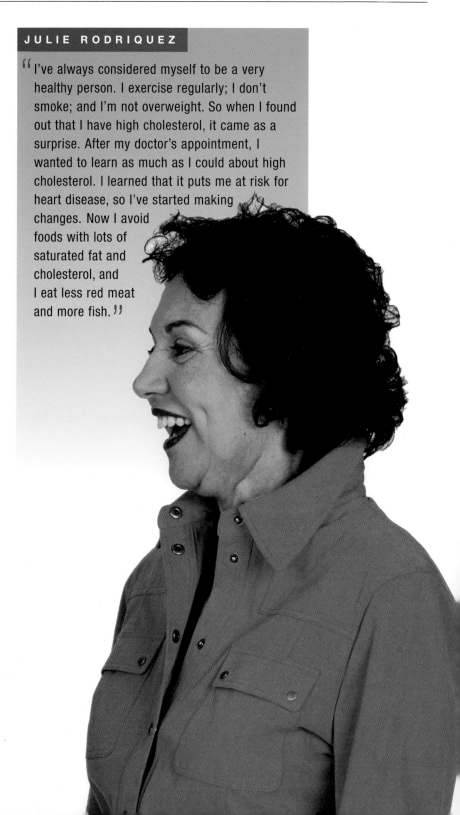

JULIE RODRIQUEZ

" I've always considered myself to be a very healthy person. I exercise regularly; I don't smoke; and I'm not overweight. So when I found out that I have high cholesterol, it came as a surprise. After my doctor's appointment, I wanted to learn as much as I could about high cholesterol. I learned that it puts me at risk for heart disease, so I've started making changes. Now I avoid foods with lots of saturated fat and cholesterol, and I eat less red meat and more fish. "

Getting Tested
High blood cholesterol itself does not cause symptoms, so if your cholesterol level is too high, you may not be aware of it. That's why it is
important to get your cholesterol levels checked regularly. Starting at
age 20, everyone should have their cholesterol levels checked by
means of a blood test called a lipoprotein profile. Be sure to ask for
the test results, so you will know whether you need to lower your
cholesterol. Ask your doctor how soon you should be retested.

Total cholesterol is a measure of the cholesterol in all of your
lipoproteins, including the "bad" cholesterol in LDL and the "good"
cholesterol in HDL. An LDL level below 100 mg/dL is considered
"optimal" or ideal. As you can see in the accompanying table, there
are four other categories of LDL levels. The higher your LDL number, the higher your risk of heart disease. Knowing your LDL number is especially important because it will determine the kind of
treatment you may need.

Your HDL number tells a different story. The lower your HDL
number, the higher your heart disease risk.

Your lipoprotein profile test will also measure levels of triglycerides,
which are another fatty substance in the blood. (See "Tame Your
Triglycerides.")

What's Your Number?

Blood Cholesterol Levels and Heart Disease Risk

Total Cholesterol Level	Category
Less than 200 mg/dL*	Desirable
200–239 mg/dL	Borderline high
240 mg/dL and above	High

LDL Cholesterol Level	Category
Less than 100 mg/dL	Optimal (ideal)
100–129 mg/dL	Nearly optimal
130–159 mg/dL	Borderline high
160–189 mg/dL	High
190 mg/dL and above	Very high

* *Cholesterol levels are measured in milligrams (mg) of cholesterol per deciliter (dL) of blood.*

Major Risk Factors

Tame Your
Triglycerides

Triglycerides are another type of fat found in blood and in food. Triglycerides are produced in the liver. When you drink alcohol or take in more calories than your body needs, your liver produces more triglycerides. Triglyceride levels that are borderline high (150–199 mg/dL) or high (200–499 mg/dL) are signals of an increased risk for heart disease. To reduce blood triglyceride levels, it is important to control your weight, get more physical activity, and avoid smoking and drinking alcohol. You should also eat a diet that is low in saturated fat, *trans* fat, and cholesterol and that avoids high amounts of carbohydrates. Sometimes, medication is needed.

Triglycerides

HDL Cholesterol Level
An HDL cholesterol level of less than 40 mg/dL is a major risk factor for heart disease. An HDL level of 60 mg/dL or higher is somewhat protective.

Heart Disease Risk and Your LDL Goal
In general, the higher your LDL cholesterol level and the more other risk factors you have, the greater your chances of developing heart disease or having a heart attack. The higher your overall risk, the lower your LDL goal level will be. Here is how to determine your LDL goal:

Step 1: Count your risk factors. Below are risk factors for heart disease that will affect your LDL goal. Check to see how many of the following risk factors[1] you have:
- Cigarette smoking
- High blood pressure (140/90 mmHg or higher, or if you are on blood pressure medication)

---

[1] *Diabetes is not on the list because a person with diabetes is considered to already be at high risk for a heart attack—at the same level of risk as someone who has heart disease. Also, even though overweight and physical inactivity are not on this list of risk factors, they are conditions that raise your risk for heart disease and need to be corrected.*

- Low HDL cholesterol (less than 40 mg/dL)[2]
- Family history of early heart disease (your father or brother before age 55, or your mother or sister before age 65)
- Age (55 or older if you're a woman; 45 or older if you're a man)

Step 2: Find out your risk score. If you have two or more risk factors on the above list, you will need to figure out your "risk score." This score will show your chances of having a heart attack within the next 10 years. To find out your risk score, see "How To Estimate Your Risk" on pages 86–87. Note that there are separate risk "scorecards" for men and women.

Step 3: Find out your risk category. Use your number of risk factors, risk score, and medical history to find out your category of risk for heart disease or heart attack. Use the table below.

If You Have	Your Category Is
Heart disease, diabetes, or a risk score of more than 20 percent*	High risk
Two or more risk factors and a risk score of 10–20 percent	Next highest risk
Two or more risk factors and a risk score of less than 10 percent	Moderate risk
Zero or one risk factor	Low-to-moderate risk

* *Means that more than 20 of 100 people in this category will have a heart attack within 10 years.*

A Special Type of Risk

Nearly 25 percent of Americans have a group of risk factors known as metabolic syndrome, which is usually caused by overweight or obesity and by not getting enough physical activity. This cluster of risk factors increases your risk of developing heart disease and

[2] *If your HDL cholesterol is 60 mg/dL or higher, subtract 1 from your total.*

diabetes, regardless of your LDL cholesterol level. You have metabolic syndrome if you have three or more of the following conditions:

- A waist measurement of 35 inches or more for a woman or 40 inches or more for a man
- Triglycerides of 150 mg/dL or more
- An HDL cholesterol level of less than 50 mg/dL for a woman and less than 40 mg/dL for a man
- Blood pressure of 130/85 mmHg or more (either number counts)
- Blood sugar of 100 mg/dL or more

If you have metabolic syndrome, you should calculate your risk score and risk category as indicated in Steps 2 and 3 above. You should make a particularly strong effort to reach and maintain your LDL goal. You should also emphasize weight control and physical activity to correct the risk factors of the metabolic syndrome.

Your LDL Goal

The main goal of cholesterol-lowering treatment is to lower your LDL level enough to reduce your risk of heart disease or heart attack. The higher your risk category, the lower your LDL goal will be. To find your personal LDL goal, see the table below:

If You Are in This Risk Category	Your LDL Goal Is
High Risk	Less than 100 mg/dL
Next highest risk or moderate risk	Less than 130 mg/dL
Low-to-moderate risk	Less than 160 mg/dL

How to Lower Your LDL

There are two main ways to lower your LDL cholesterol—through lifestyle changes alone, or through lifestyle changes combined with medication. Depending on your risk category, the use of these treatments will differ.

For information on the best treatment plan for your risk category, see the factsheet, "High Blood Cholesterol: What You Need To Know," available from NHLBI's Web site or Health Information Center. (See "To Learn More" on page 88.)

Cholesterol-
Lowering Medicine

As part of your cholesterol-lowering treatment plan, your doctor may recommend medication. You may be prescribed just one cholesterol-lowering drug, or two in combination. Following are the most commonly used medicines:

Statins. These are the most commonly prescribed drugs for people who need a cholesterol-lowering medicine. Of all available medications, statins lower LDL cholesterol the most, usually by 20 to 60 percent. Side effects are usually mild, although liver and muscle problems occur rarely. If you experience muscle aches or weakness, contact your doctor promptly.

Bile acid sequestrants. These medications lower LDL cholesterol by about 10 to 20 percent. Bile acid sequestrants are often prescribed along with a statin to further decrease LDL cholesterol levels. Side effects may include constipation, bloating, nausea, and gas. However, long-term use of these medicines is considered safe.

Niacin. Niacin, or nicotinic acid, lowers total cholesterol, LDL cholesterol, and triglyceride levels, while also raising HDL cholesterol. Niacin is available without a prescription, but it is important to use it only under a doctor's care because of possible serious side effects. In some people, it may worsen peptic ulcers or cause liver problems, gout, or high blood sugar.

Fibrates. These drugs can reduce triglycerides levels by 20 to 50 percent, while increasing HDL cholesterol by 10 to 15 percent. Fibrates are not very effective for lowering LDL cholesterol. The drugs can increase the chances of developing gallstones and heighten the effects of blood-thinning drugs.

Ezetimibe. This is the first in a new class of cholesterol-lowering drugs that interfere with the absorption of cholesterol in the intestine. It can be used alone or in combination with a statin. Side effects may include back and joint pain.

Lifestyle changes. One important treatment approach is called TLC, which stands for "Therapeutic Lifestyle Changes." This treatment includes a low saturated fat and low-cholesterol diet, regular moderate-intensity physical activity, and weight management. Everyone who needs to lower their LDL cholesterol should use this TLC program. (For more information, see "Give Your Heart a Little TLC" on page 55.) Maintaining a healthy weight and getting regular physical activity are especially important for those who have metabolic syndrome.

Medication. If your LDL level stays too high even after making lifestyle changes, you may need to take medicine. If you need medication, be sure to use it along with the TLC approach. This will keep the dose of medicine as low as possible, and will lower your risk in other ways as well. You will also need to control all of your other heart disease risk factors, including high blood pressure, diabetes, and smoking.

Overweight and Obesity

A healthy weight is important for a long, vigorous life. Yet overweight and obesity (extreme overweight) have reached epidemic levels in the United States. Today, nearly two-thirds of American adults are overweight or obese. Groups at highest risk for obesity include African American women, Mexican Americans, and American Indians, but millions of people from all backgrounds weigh more than is healthy for them. Since 1991, the proportion of Americans who are obese has soared by 75 percent.

Overweight among children is also swiftly increasing. Among young people ages 6–19, more than 16 percent are overweight, compared to just 4 percent a few decades ago. This is a disturbing trend because overweight adolescents have a greatly increased risk of dying from heart disease in adulthood. Even our youngest citizens are at risk. About 10 percent of preschoolers weigh more than is healthy for them.

Our national waistline is expanding for two simple reasons—we are eating more and moving less. Americans consume about 200–300 more calories per day than they did in the 1970s. Moreover, as we spend more time in front of computers, video games, TV, and other electronic pastimes, we have fewer hours available for physical activity.

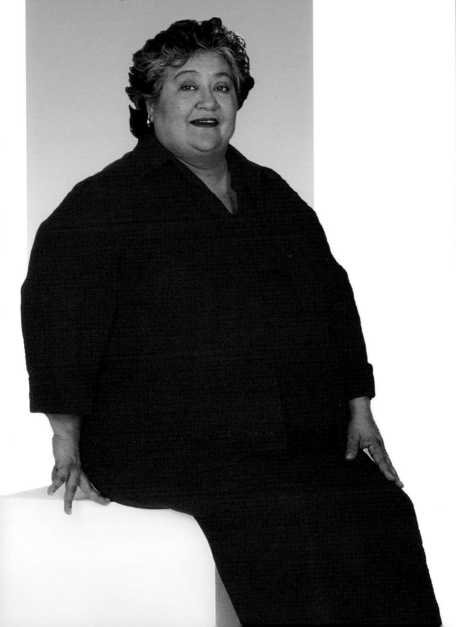

BALERMA BURGESS

"I know that if I don't change things in my life, I might not live to see my grandchildren. Every day, I talk myself into doing things for my health, like taking the stairs instead of the elevator and eating more fruits and vegetables. These things haven't become habits for me yet, but I'm working on it."

There is growing evidence of a link between "couch potato" behavior and increased risk of obesity and many chronic diseases.

It is hard to overstate the dangers of an unhealthy weight. If you are overweight, you are more likely to develop heart disease even if you have no other risk factors. The more overweight a person is, the more likely he or she is to develop heart disease. Overweight and obesity also increase the risks for diabetes, high blood pressure, high cholesterol, stroke, congestive heart failure, gallbladder disease, arthritis, breathing problems, and gout, as well as cancers of the breast and colon. Each year, an estimated 300,000 U.S. adults die of diseases related to obesity. The bottom line: Maintaining a healthy weight is a vital part of preventing heart disease and protecting overall health.

Should You Choose To Lose?

Do you need to lose weight to reduce your risk of heart disease? You can find out by taking three simple steps.

Step 1: Get your number. Take a look at the box on the next page. You'll see that your weight in relation to your height gives you a number called a Body Mass Index (BMI). A BMI from 18.5 to 24.9 indicates a normal weight. A person with a BMI from 25 to 29.9 is overweight, while someone with a BMI of 30 or higher is obese. Those in the overweight and obese categories have a higher risk of heart disease—and the higher the BMI, the greater the risk.

Step 2: Take out a tape measure. The second step is to take your waist measurement. For women, a waist measurement of over 35 inches increases the risk of heart disease as well as the risks of high blood pressure, diabetes, and other serious health conditions. For men, a waist measurement of more than 40 inches increases these risks. To measure your waist correctly, stand and place a tape measure around your middle, just above your hipbones. Measure your waist just after you breathe out.

Step 3: Review your risk. The final step in determining your need to lose weight is to find out your other risk factors for heart disease. It is important to know whether you have any of the following: high blood pressure, high LDL cholesterol, low HDL cholesterol, high triglycerides, high blood glucose (blood sugar), a family history of heart disease, physical inactivity, or smoking. If you're a man,

Are You at a Healthy Weight?

Here is a chart for men and women that gives the BMI for various heights and weights*

BODY MASS INDEX

	21	22	23	24	25	26	27	28	29	30	31
4'10"	100	105	110	115	119	124	129	134	138	143	148
5'0"	107	112	118	123	128	133	138	143	148	153	158
5'1"	111	116	122	127	132	137	143	148	153	158	164
5'3"	118	124	130	135	141	146	152	158	163	169	175
5'5"	126	132	138	144	150	156	162	168	174	180	186
5'7"	134	140	146	153	159	166	172	178	185	191	198
5'9"	142	149	155	162	169	176	182	189	196	203	209
5'11"	150	157	165	172	179	186	193	200	208	215	222
6'1"	159	166	174	182	189	197	204	212	219	227	235
6'3"	168	176	184	192	200	208	216	224	232	240	248

* Weight is measured with underwear but not shoes.

What Does Your BMI Mean?

Categories:

Normal weight: BMI = 18.5–24.9. Good for you! Try not to gain weight.

Overweight: BMI = 25–29.9. Do not gain any weight, especially if your waist measurement is high. You need to lose weight if you have two or more risk factors for heart disease and are overweight, or have a high waist measurement.

Obese: BMI = 30 or greater. You need to lose weight. Lose weight slowly—about 1/2 to 2 pounds a week. See your doctor or nutritionist if you need help.

Source: Clinical Guidelines on the Identification, Evaluation and Treatment of Overweight and Obesity in Adults: The Evidence Report; National Heart, Lung, and Blood Institute, in cooperation with the National Institute of Diabetes and Digestive and Kidney Diseases, National Institutes of Health; NIH Publication 98-4083; June 1998.

Major Risk Factors

Keeping Tabs on Your Progress

You can reduce your risk of heart disease. Set goals for blood pressure, cholesterol, and weight with your doctor. If you have diabetes, also set goals for blood glucose (or blood sugar) levels. Fill out the important information below each time you get your cholesterol or blood pressure measured, or get other measurements.

Blood Pressure

Date	Blood Pressure
	/
	/

My Goal Blood Pressure: _____

Cholesterol

Date	Total	LDL	HDL

My Goal LDL: _____

Triglyceride levels can also raise heart disease risk. Levels that are borderline high (150–199 mg/dL) or high (200 mg/dL or more) may need treatment in some people.

Blood Glucose

Date	Blood Glucose Level

My Goal Blood Glucose Level: _____

Weight

Date	Weight	Body Mass Index (BMI)

My Goal Weight: _____ My Goal BMI: _____

Blood Pressure

Normal:	less than 120/80 mmHg
Prehypertension:	120/80 to 139/89 mmHg
Hypertension:	140/90 or higher mmHg

Cholesterol

Total Cholesterol

Desirable:	less than 200 mg/dL
Borderline high:	200–239 mg/dL
High:	240 mg/dL and above

LDL Cholesterol

Optimal	less than 100 mg/dL
Near optimal	100–129 mg/dL
Borderline high	130–159 mg/dL
High	160–189 mg/dL
Very high	190 mg/dL and above

HDL Cholesterol

An HDL cholesterol of less than 40 mg/dL is a major risk factor for heart disease.

Blood Glucose

Normal:	under 99 mg/dL
Prediabetes:	100–125 mg/dL
Diabetes:	126 mg/dL and above

BMI

Normal weight:	BMI = 18.5–24.9
Overweight:	BMI = 25–29.9
Obese:	BMI = 30 or greater

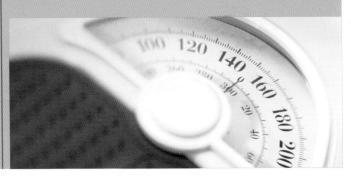

being age 45 or older is also a heart disease risk factor. For a woman, being age 55 or older or having gone through menopause increases the risk. If you have a condition known as metabolic syndrome, your risk of heart disease is increased. (See "A Special Type of Risk" on page 21.) If you aren't sure whether you have some of these risk factors, ask your doctor.

Once you've taken these three steps, you can use the information to decide if you need to take off pounds. While you should talk with your doctor about whether you should lose weight, keep these guidelines in mind:

- If you are overweight AND have two or more other risk factors, or if you are obese, you should lose weight.
- If you are overweight, have a high waist measurement (over 35 inches for a woman; over 40 inches for a man), AND have two or more other risk factors, you should lose weight.
- If you are overweight, but do not have a high waist measurement and have fewer than two other risk factors, you should avoid further weight gain.

Lose a Little, Win a Lot

If you need to lose weight, here's some good news: A small weight loss—just 5 to 10 percent of your current weight—will help to lower your risk for heart disease and other serious medical disorders. The best way to take off pounds is to do so gradually by getting regular physical activity and eating a balanced diet that is lower in calories and saturated fat. For some people at very high risk, medication also may be necessary. To develop a weight-loss or weight-mainte-nance program that works well for you, consult with your doctor, registered dietitian, or qualified nutritionist. For ideas on how to lose weight safely and keep it off, see "Aim for a Healthy Weight" on page 61.

Physical Inactivity

"I'd love to take a walk—tomorrow."
"I can't wait to start yoga—if I can find a good class."
"I'm going to start lifting weights—as soon as I get the time."

Many of us put off getting regular physical activity, and hope that our bodies will understand. But our bodies *don't* understand, and sooner or later, they rebel. Even if a person has no other risk factors, being physically inactive greatly boosts the chances of developing heart-related problems. It also increases the likelihood of developing other heart disease risk factors, such as high blood pressure, diabetes, and overweight. Lack of physical activity also leads to more visits to the doctor, more hospitalizations, and more use of medicines for a variety of illnesses.

Despite these risks, most Americans aren't getting enough physical activity. According to the CDC, nearly 40 percent of Americans are not active at all during their free time. Overall, women tend to be less physically active than men, and older people are less likely to be active than younger individuals. But young people need to get moving, too. Forty percent of high school-aged girls and 27 percent of high school-aged boys don't get enough physical activity to protect their health.

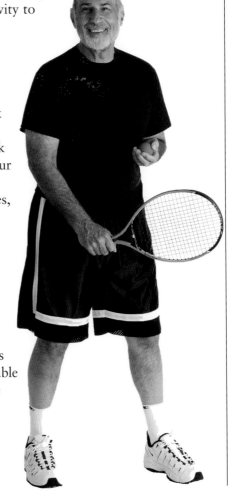

Fortunately, research shows that as little as 30 minutes of moderate-intensity physical activity on most, and preferably all, days of the week helps to protect heart health. This level of activity can reduce your risk of heart disease as well as lower your chances of having a stroke, colon cancer, high blood pressure, diabetes, and other medical problems.

Examples of moderate activity are taking a brisk walk, light weight-lifting, dancing, raking leaves, washing a car, house cleaning, or gardening. If you prefer, you can divide your 30-minute activity into shorter periods of at least 10 minutes each. To find out about easy, enjoyable ways to boost your activity level, see "Get Moving!" on page 72.

Diabetes

Diabetes is a major risk factor for heart disease and stroke. More than 65 percent of people who have diabetes die of some type of cardiovascular disease. Diabetic women are at especially high risk for dying of heart disease and stroke. Today, about 14 million people in the United States have diagnosed diabetes. In addition, nearly 6 million people have this serious disease but don't know it.

The type of diabetes that most commonly develops in adulthood is type 2 diabetes. In type 2 diabetes, the pancreas makes insulin, but the body cannot use it properly and gradually loses the ability to produce it. Type 2 diabetes is a serious disease. In addition to increasing the risk for heart disease, it is the #1 cause of kidney failure, blindness, and lower limb amputation in adults. Diabetes can also lead to nerve damage and difficulties with fighting infection.

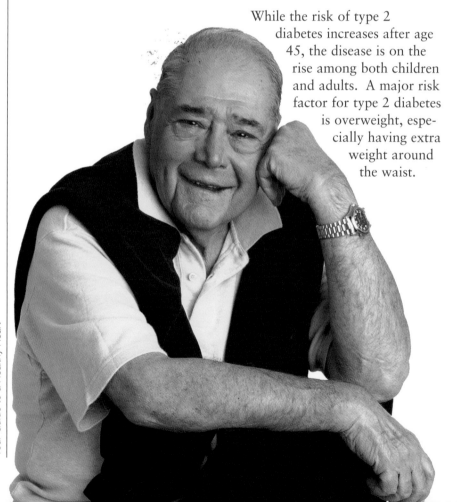

While the risk of type 2 diabetes increases after age 45, the disease is on the rise among both children and adults. A major risk factor for type 2 diabetes is overweight, especially having extra weight around the waist.

Other risk factors include physical inactivity and a family history of diabetes. Type 2 diabetes also is more common among American Indians, Hispanic Americans, African Americans, Asian Americans, and Pacific Islanders. Women who have had diabetes during pregnancy (gestational diabetes) or have given birth to a baby weighing more than 9 pounds are also more likely to develop type 2 diabetes later in life.

Symptoms of diabetes may include fatigue, nausea, frequent urination, unusual thirst, weight loss, blurred vision, frequent infections, and slow healing of sores. But type 2 diabetes develops gradually and sometimes has no symptoms. Even if you have no symptoms of diabetes, if you are overweight and have any of the risk factors for type 2 diabetes, ask your doctor about getting tested for it. You have diabetes if your fasting blood glucose level is 126 mg/dL or higher.

If you have diabetes, controlling your blood glucose (blood sugar) levels will help to prevent complications. Because diabetes is so strongly linked with heart disease, managing diabetes must include keeping certain factors under control. (See "The ABCs of Diabetes Control.") Recommended levels of blood pressure and blood cholesterol control are lower for people with diabetes than for most others. Not smoking, being physically active, and taking aspirin daily (if your doctor recommends it) also are important ways to prevent heart disease if you have diabetes.

Some people do not yet have diabetes, but are at high risk for developing the disease. More than 14 million Americans have a condition known as "prediabetes," in which blood glucose levels are higher than normal but not yet in the diabetic range. Prediabetes is defined as a fasting blood glucose level of 100–125 mg/dL. New research shows that many people with prediabetes can prevent or delay the development of diabetes by making modest changes in diet and level of physical activity. (See "Preventing Diabetes.")

People who are prediabetic also have a 50 percent greater chance of having a heart attack or stroke than those with normal blood glucose levels. If you are prediabetic, you'll need to pay close attention to preventing or controlling high blood pressure, high blood cholesterol, and other risk factors for heart disease.

The ABCs of
Diabetes Control

If you have diabetes, three key steps can help you lower your risk of heart attack and stroke. Follow these ABCs:

A **is for A1C test,** which is short for hemoglobin A1C. This test measures your average blood glucose over the last 3 months. It lets you know if your blood glucose level is under control. Get this test at least twice a year. Number to aim for: below 7.

B **is for blood pressure.** The higher your blood pressure, the harder your heart has to work. Get your blood pressure measured at every doctor's visit. Numbers to aim for: below 130/80 mmHg.

C **is for cholesterol.** LDL, or "bad" cholesterol, builds up and clogs your arteries. Get your LDL cholesterol tested at least once a year. Number to aim for: below 100 mg/dL. If you have both diabetes and heart disease, your doctor may advise you to aim for a lower target number, for example, less than 70.

Be sure to ask your doctor:
1. What are my ABC numbers?
2. What should my ABC target numbers be?
3. What actions should I take to reach my ABC target numbers?

To lower your risk of heart attack and stroke, also take these steps:
- Be physically active every day.
- Follow your doctor's advice about getting physical activity every day.
- Eat less salt and sodium, saturated fat, *trans* fat, and cholesterol.
- Eat more fiber. Choose fiber-rich whole grains, fruits, vegetables, and beans.
- Stay at a healthy weight.
- If you smoke, stop.
- Take medicines as prescribed.
- Ask your doctor about taking aspirin.
- Ask others to help you manage your diabetes.

Preventing
Diabetes

If you have "prediabetes"—higher than normal glucose levels—you are more likely to develop type 2 diabetes. But you can take steps to improve your health, and delay or possibly prevent diabetes. A recent study showed that many overweight, prediabetic people dramatically reduced their risk of developing diabetes by following a lower fat, lower calorie diet and getting 30 minutes of physical activity at least 5 days per week. The following are some encouraging results of the study:

- Overall, people who achieved a 5- to 7-percent weight loss (about 10 to 15 pounds) through diet and increased physical activity (usually brisk walking) reduced their risk of diabetes by 58 percent over the next 3 years.
- For people over age 60, these lifestyle changes reduced the risk of developing diabetes by 71 percent.
- Benefits were seen in all of the racial and ethnic groups that participated in the study—White, African American, Hispanic, American Indian, Asian American, and Pacific Islanders.
- People taking the diabetes drug metformin (Glucophage) reduced their risk of developing the disease by 31 percent.

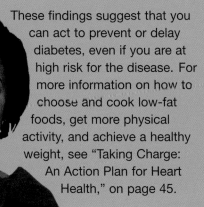

These findings suggest that you can act to prevent or delay diabetes, even if you are at high risk for the disease. For more information on how to choose and cook low-fat foods, get more physical activity, and achieve a healthy weight, see "Taking Charge: An Action Plan for Heart Health," on page 45.

Major Risk Factors

What Else Affects Heart Disease?

A number of other factors affect heart disease, including certain health conditions, medicines, and other substances. Here is what you need to know:

Stress
Stress is linked to heart disease in a number of ways. Research shows that the most commonly reported "trigger" for a heart attack is an emotionally upsetting event, particularly one involving anger. In addition, some common ways of coping with stress, such as overeating, heavy drinking, and smoking, are clearly bad for your heart. The good news is that sensible health habits can have a protective effect. Regular physical activity not only relieves stress, but also can directly lower your risk of heart disease. Stress management programs can also help you develop new ways of handling everyday life challenges. Good relationships count, too. Developing strong personal ties reduces the chances of developing heart disease.

Much remains to be learned about the connections between stress and heart disease, but a few things are clear. Staying physically active, developing a wide circle of supportive people in your life, and sharing your feelings and concerns with them can help you be happier and live longer.

Alcohol
Recent research suggests that moderate drinkers are less likely to develop heart disease than people who don't drink any alcohol or who drink too much. Small amounts of alcohol may help protect against heart disease by raising levels of HDL "good" cholesterol.

If you are a nondrinker, this is *not* a recommendation to start using alcohol. If you are a pregnant woman, if you're planning to become pregnant, or if you have another health condition that could make alcohol use harmful, you should not drink. Otherwise, if you're already a moderate drinker, you may be less likely to have a heart attack.

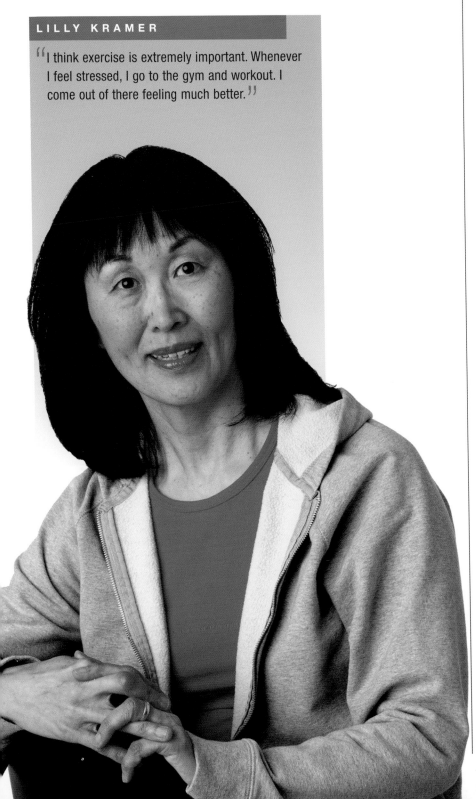

LILLY KRAMER

"I think exercise is extremely important. Whenever I feel stressed, I go to the gym and workout. I come out of there feeling much better."

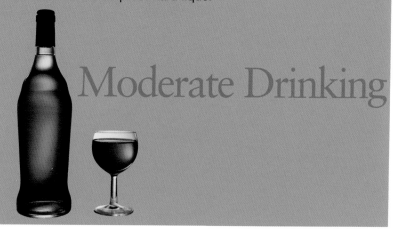

What Is Moderate Drinking?

Moderate drinking is defined as no more than one drink per day for women, and no more than two drinks per day for men, according to the "U.S. Dietary Guidelines for Americans." Count as one drink:

- 12 ounces of beer
- 5 ounces of wine
- 1½ ounces of 80-proof hard liquor

It is important, though, to weigh benefits against risks. Talk with your doctor about your personal risks of heart disease and other health conditions that may be affected by drinking alcohol. With the help of your doctor, decide whether moderate drinking to lower heart attack risk outweighs the possible increased risk of other medical problems.

If you do decide to use alcohol, remember that moderation is the key. Heavy drinking causes many heart-related problems. More than three drinks per day can raise blood pressure and triglyceride levels, while binge drinking can contribute to stroke. Too much alcohol also can damage the heart muscle, leading to heart failure. Overall, people who drink heavily on a regular basis have higher rates of heart disease than either moderate drinkers or nondrinkers.

Sleep Apnea

Sleep apnea is a serious disorder in which a person briefly and repeatedly stops breathing during sleep. People with untreated sleep apnea are more likely to develop high blood pressure, heart attack, congestive heart failure, and stroke.

Sleep apnea tends to develop in middle age, and men are twice as likely as women to have the condition. Other factors that increase risk are overweight and obesity, smoking, using alcohol or sleeping pills, and a family history of sleep apnea. Symptoms include heavy snoring and gasping or choking during sleep, along with extreme daytime sleepiness.

If you think you might have sleep apnea, ask your doctor for a test called a polysomnography, which is usually performed overnight in a sleep center. If you are overweight, even a small weight loss—10 percent of your current weight—can relieve mild cases of sleep apnea. Other self-help treatments include quitting smoking and avoiding alcohol and sleeping pills. Sleeping on your side rather than on your back also may help. Some people benefit from a mechanical device that helps maintain a regular breathing pattern by increasing air pressure through the nasal passages via a face mask. For very serious cases, surgery may be needed.

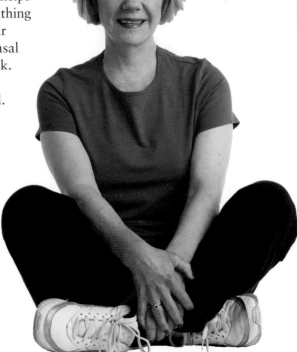

Menopausal Hormone Therapy

Until recently, it was thought that menopausal hormone therapy could ward off heart disease, osteoporosis, and cancer, as well as improve a woman's quality of life. But several important studies, conducted as part of the Women's Health Initiative, show that long-term use of hormone therapy poses serious health risks, including increased risks of heart attack, stroke, and a condition called venous thrombosis (a blood clot that usually occurs in one of the deep veins of the leg).

In one study, 16,608 postmenopausal women with a uterus took either estrogen-plus-progestin therapy or a placebo—a pill that looks like the real drug but has no biological effect. The results were surprising: The estrogen-plus-progestin therapy actually *increased* women's risk for heart attacks, stroke, blood clots, and breast cancer. A related study showed that the hormone combination doubled the risk of dementia and failed to protect women from memory loss. However, the estrogen-plus-progestin medication did reduce the risks of both colorectal cancer and bone fractures. It also relieved menopausal symptoms such as hot flashes and night sweats.

The second study involved 10,739 women who had had a hysterectomy and took either estrogen alone or a placebo. The results: Estrogen-alone therapy increased the risks for both stroke and venous thrombosis. The treatment had no effect on heart disease and colorectal cancer, and an uncertain effect on breast cancer. Estrogen alone offered no protection against memory loss. Estrogen alone, however, did reduce the risk for bone fractures.

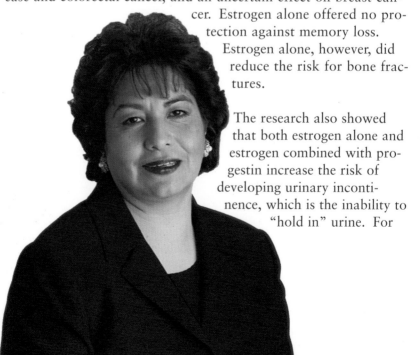

The research also showed that both estrogen alone and estrogen combined with progestin increase the risk of developing urinary incontinence, which is the inability to "hold in" urine. For women who already have the condition, these medications can worsen symptoms.

If you are a woman who is taking menopausal hormone therapy, or if you've used it in the past, these findings can't help but concern you. It's important to understand, however, that the results apply to a very large group of women. For an individual woman, the increased risk for disease is quite small. For example, in the estrogen-plus-progestin study, each woman had an increased risk of breast cancer of less than one-tenth of 1 percent per year.

While questions remain, these findings provide a basis for advice about using hormone therapy:

- Estrogen alone, or estrogen-plus-progestin, should not be used to prevent heart disease. Talk with your doctor about other ways of preventing heart attack and stroke, including lifestyle changes and medicines such as cholesterol-lowering statins and blood pressure drugs.
- If you are considering using menopausal hormone therapy to prevent the bone-thinning disease osteoporosis, talk with your doctor about the possible benefits weighed against your personal risks for heart attack, stroke, blood clots, and breast cancer. Ask your doctor about alternative treatments that are safe and effective in preventing osteoporosis and bone fractures.
- Do not take menopausal hormone therapy to prevent dementia or memory loss.
- If you are considering menopausal hormone therapy to provide relief from menopausal symptoms such as hot flashes, talk with your doctor about whether this treatment is right for you. The studies did not test the short-term risks and benefits of using hormone therapy for menopausal symptoms. The U.S. Food and Drug Administration recommends that menopausal hormone therapy be used at the lowest dose for the shortest period of time to reach treatment goals.

Remember, your risks for heart disease, stroke, osteoporosis, and other conditions may change as you age, so review your health needs regularly with your doctor. New treatments that are safe and effective may become available. Stay informed.

What Else Affects Heart Disease?

New **Risk Factors?**

We know that major risk factors such as high blood cholesterol, high blood pressure, and smoking boost heart disease risk. Researchers are studying other factors that might contribute to heart disease, including inflammation of the artery walls. Several emerging risk factors have been identified. We don't know for sure yet whether they lead to heart disease or whether treating them will reduce risk. While these possible risk factors are not recommended for routine testing, ask your doctor whether you should be tested for any of them.

C-reactive protein (CRP). High levels of CRP may indicate inflammation in the artery walls. A simple blood test can measure the levels of CRP in the blood. In many cases, a high CRP level is a sign of metabolic syndrome. Treatment of the syndrome with lifestyle changes—weight loss and regular physical activity—can often lower CRP.

Homocysteine. High blood levels of this amino acid may increase risk for heart disease. It may be possible to lower elevated levels of homocysteine by getting plenty of folic acid and vitamins B6 and B12 in your diet.

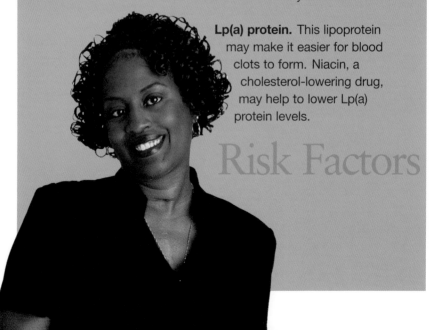

Lp(a) protein. This lipoprotein may make it easier for blood clots to form. Niacin, a cholesterol-lowering drug, may help to lower Lp(a) protein levels.

Risk Factors

Birth Control Pills

Studies show that women who use high-dose birth control pills (oral contraceptives) are more likely to have a heart attack or stroke because blood clots are more likely to form in the blood vessels. These risks are lessened once the birth control pill is stopped. Using the pill also may worsen the effects of other risk factors, such as smoking, high blood pressure, diabetes, high blood cholesterol, and overweight.

Much of this information comes from studies of birth control pills containing higher doses of hormones than those commonly used today. Still, the risks of using low-dose pills are not fully known. Therefore, if you are now taking any kind of birth control pill or are considering using one, keep these guidelines in mind:

Don't mix smoking and the "pill." If you smoke cigarettes, stop smoking or choose a different form of birth control. Cigarette smoking raises the risk of serious health problems from birth control pill use, especially the risk of blood clots. For women over 35, the risk is particularly high. Women who use birth control pills should not smoke.

Pay attention to diabetes. Levels of glucose, or blood sugar, sometimes change dramatically in women who take birth control pills. If you are diabetic or have a close relative who is, be sure to have regular blood sugar tests if you take birth control pills.

Watch your blood pressure. After starting to take birth control pills, your blood pressure may go up. If your blood pressure increases to 140/90 mmHg or higher, ask your doctor about changing pills or switching to another form of birth control. Be sure to get your blood pressure checked at least once a year.

Talk with your doctor. If you have heart disease or another heart problem, or if you have suffered a stroke, birth control pills may not be a safe choice. Be sure your doctor knows about these and any other serious health conditions before prescribing birth control pills for you.

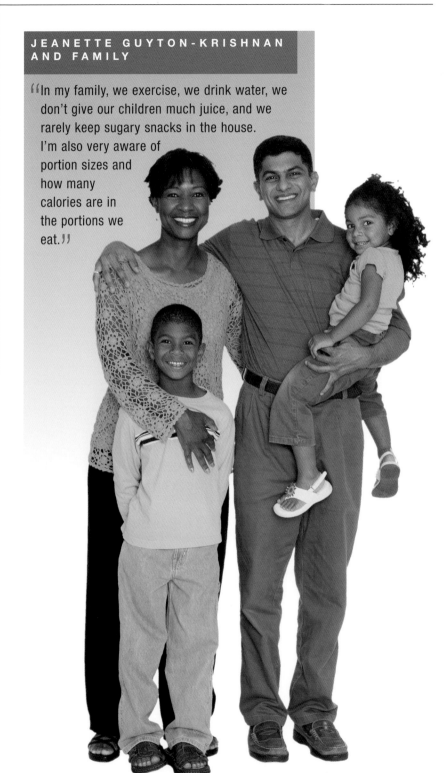

JEANETTE GUYTON-KRISHNAN AND FAMILY

"In my family, we exercise, we drink water, we don't give our children much juice, and we rarely keep sugary snacks in the house. I'm also very aware of portion sizes and how many calories are in the portions we eat."

Taking Charge: An Action Plan for Heart Health

You have just learned a great deal about risk factors for heart disease. Now you're ready for action. The good news: Research shows that people can lower their heart disease risk enormously— by as much as 82 percent—simply by adopting sensible health habits. It's never too late to start protecting your heart health. A recent study shows that among people ages 70 to 90, leading a healthy lifestyle reduces the chances of dying from heart disease by nearly two-thirds.

What does it mean to "lead a healthy lifestyle"? Here are the basics: If you eat a nutritious diet, get regular physical activity, maintain a healthy weight, and stop smoking, you will help to keep your heart healthy. But doing just one or two of these "Big Four" habits isn't enough to protect your heart. To keep your heart strong and healthy, it is vital to adopt and practice all four lifestyle habits.

Some people may need to take additional steps to prevent heart disease. For example, if you have diabetes, you also will need to keep your blood sugar levels under control. Eating a nutritious diet, controlling your weight, and getting more physical activity will help you to keep your blood sugar at healthy levels. These steps will also help reduce your chances of developing high blood pressure or high blood cholesterol. Whatever your current health condition or habits, the action plan that follows will make a positive difference in your heart health.

Ready to get started? Read on.

Choose Healthy Foods

A healthy heart needs a healthy diet. The "Dietary Guidelines for Americans" offers two examples of eating plans to choose from, and also includes advice for overall health and food safety. These guide-lines encourage you to:

- Choose a variety of grains daily; half of your daily grains should come from whole grains.
- Choose a variety of fruits and vegetables daily.
- Choose a diet that is low in saturated fat, *trans* fat, and cholesterol.
- Choose foods and beverages that are low in added sugar.
- Choose and prepare foods with little salt.
- If you drink alcoholic beverages, do so in moderation.
- Aim for a healthy weight.
- Be physically active most days.
- Balance the calories you take in with the calories you expend through physical activity.
- Keep foods safe to eat.

For detailed tips on getting regular physical activity and maintaining a healthy weight, see later sections of this guidebook.

Getting Extra Support

While the "Dietary Guidelines for Americans" offer an excellent "basic menu" for heart health, you may need to make some additional changes in your diet if you have high blood pressure or high

What Are *Trans* Fats?

Trans fats, or *trans* fatty acids, are another type of dietary fat that raises LDL cholesterol. They are formed when vegetable oil is hardened to become margarine or shortening in a process called hydrogenation. The harder the margarine or shortening, the more likely it is to contain more *trans* fat. To reduce *trans* fats in your diet, read food labels and buy fewer products that list "hydrogenated oil" or "partially hydrogenated oil" as an ingredient. When possible, choose margarines that list "liquid vegetable oil" as the first ingredient. The main sources of *trans* fat are foods made with hydrogenated oils such as some margarines, shortenings, cookies, crackers, cakes, pies, snack foods, and fried foods.

Trans Fats

How To Use the
Nutrition Facts Label
on the Food Package

Start here

Check calories

Limit these nutrients

Get enough of these nutrients

Nutrition Facts

Serving Size 1 cup (228g)
Servings Per Container 2

Amount Per Serving

Calories 250	Calories from Fat 110

	% Daily Value*
Total Fat 12g	**18%**
Saturated Fat 3g	**15%**
Trans Fat 3g	
Cholesterol 30mg	**10%**
Sodium 470mg	**20%**
Total Carbohydrate 31g	**10%**
Dietary Fiber 0g	**0%**
Sugars 5g	
Protein 5g	

Vitamin A	4%
Vitamin C	2%
Calcium	20%
Iron	4%

* Percent Daily Values are based on a 2,000 calorie diet. Your Daily values may be higher or lower depending on your calorie needs.

	Calories:	2,000	2,500
Total Fat	Less Than	65g	80g
Sat Fat	Less Than	20g	25g
Cholesteral	Less Than	300mg	300mg
Sodium	Less than	2,400mg	2,400mg
Total Carbohydrate		300g	375g
Dietary Fiber		25g	30g

Quick Guide to % DV:
5% or less is low
20% or more is high

Nutrition Facts Label

blood cholesterol. You may want to work with a registered dietitian to help you make these changes. A dietitian can teach you about the eating plan that is best for you, determine a reasonable calorie level, and help you choose foods and plan menus. A dietitian can also help you keep track of your progress and encourage you to stay on your eating plan. Talk with your doctor about whether you should get a referral to a registered dietitian. In the meantime, if you have high blood pressure or high blood cholesterol, here are some guidelines:

Blood Pressure and the DASH Eating Plan
If you have high blood pressure or prehypertension, you may want to follow an eating plan called DASH. DASH stands for "Dietary Approaches to Stop Hypertension," and the eating plan emphasizes fruits, vegetables, whole-grain foods, and low-fat milk products. It is rich in magnesium, potassium, calcium, protein, and fiber, but low in saturated fat, *trans* fat, total fat, and cholesterol. It limits red meat, sweets, and beverages with added sugars. In many ways, DASH is similar to the TLC eating plan described on pages 53–55. However, the DASH plan also encourages you to eat specific foods rich in the nutrients noted above.

A major study found that people who followed this eating plan reduced their blood pressure more than those who ate more "typical" American diets, which have fewer fruits and vegetables. A second study found that people who followed the DASH eating plan *and* cut down on sodium had the biggest reductions in blood pressure. (Salt, or sodium chloride, and other forms of sodium are found in many processed foods. Often, more salt is added to food during cooking and at the table.) So, for a truly winning combination, follow the DASH eating plan and lower your sodium intake as much as possible. The study found that the less sodium people consumed, the more their blood pressure dropped. (See "The DASH Eating Plan" on pages 51–52 and "Please *Don't* Pass the Salt" on page 52.)

While the DASH eating plan is geared especially toward people with high blood pressure or prehypertension, it is a healthy plan for everyone. So share it with your family. When people with normal blood pressure follow the DASH eating plan, especially when they also consume less sodium, they lessen their chances of developing high blood pressure. Remember, 90 percent of middle-aged Americans go on to develop high blood pressure. Use the DASH plan to help beat the odds!

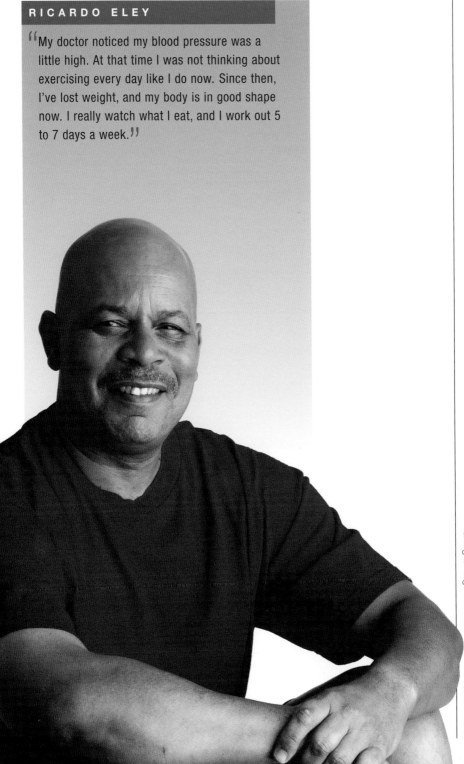

RICARDO ELEY

"My doctor noticed my blood pressure was a little high. At that time I was not thinking about exercising every day like I do now. Since then, I've lost weight, and my body is in good shape now. I really watch what I eat, and I work out 5 to 7 days a week."

The **DASH** Eating Plan

The DASH eating plan shown in the following table is based on 2,000 calories per day. The number of daily servings in a food group may vary from those listed, depending on how many daily calories you need. If you need to lose weight, you can follow the DASH eating plan and simply decrease calories by choosing fewer servings or smaller serving sizes of the foods shown on the list.

Food Group	Serving Sizes	Examples
Grain and grain products 7–8 daily servings	1 slice whole-grain bread 1 cup ready-to-eat cereal*, ½ cup cooked rice, pasta, or cereal	Whole-wheat bread, English muffin, pita bread, bagel, cereals, grits, oatmeal, crackers, unsalted pretzels, popcorn
Vegetables 4–5 daily servings	1 cup raw, dark green, leafy vegetable, ½ cup cooked vegetables, 6 ounces vegetable juice	Tomatoes, potatoes, carrots, green peas, squash, broccoli, turnip greens, collards, kale, spinach, artichokes, green beans, lima beans, sweet potatoes
Fruits 4–5 daily servings	1 medium-sized fruit ¼ cup dried fruit, ½ cup fresh, frozen, or canned fruit, 6 ounces fruit juice	Apricots, bananas, dates, grapes, oranges, orange juice, grapefruit, grapefruit juice, mangoes, melons, peaches, pineapples, prunes, raisins, strawberries, tangerines

Low-fat or fat-free milk products 2–3 daily servings	8 ounces milk, 1 cup yogurt, 1½ ounces cheese	Low-fat or fat-free milk, low-fat or fat-free buttermilk, low-fat or fat-free regular or frozen yogurt, low-fat or fat-free cheese
Lean meats, poultry, and fish 2 or fewer daily	3 ounces cooked lean meat, skinless poultry, or fish	Select only lean; trim away visible fats; broil, roast, or boil, instead of frying; remove skin from poultry
Nuts, seeds, and dry beans 4–5 servings per week	½ cup or 1½ ounces nuts, 1 tablespoon or ½ ounce seeds, ½ cup cooked dry beans	Almonds, filberts, mixed nuts, peanuts, walnuts, sunflower seeds, kidney beans, lentils
Fats and oils† 2–3 daily servings	1 teaspoon soft margarine, 1 tablespoon low-fat mayonnaise, 2 tablespoons light salad dressing, 1 teaspoon vegetable oil	Soft margarine, low-fat mayonnaise, light salad dressing, vegetable oil, such as olive, corn, canola, or safflower
Sweets 5 servings per week	1 tablespoon sugar, 1 tablespoon jelly or jam, ½ ounce jelly beans, 8 ounces lemonade	Maple syrup, sugar, jelly, jam, fruit-flavored gelatin, jelly beans, hard candy, fruit punch, sorbet, ices

* *Serving sizes vary between ½ –1¼ cups. Check the Nutrition Facts label on the product's package.*
† *Fat content changes serving counts for fats and oils. For example, 1 tablespoon of regular salad dressing equals 1 serving; 1 tablespoon of a low-fat dressing equals ½ serving; 1 tablespoon of a fat-free dressing equals 0 servings.*

Taking Charge: An Action Plan for Heart Health

Please *Don't* Pass the Salt:
How To Reduce Salt and Sodium in Your Diet

You can help prevent and control high blood pressure by cutting down on salt and other forms of sodium. Try to consume no more than 2,300 mg of sodium (approximately 1 teaspoon of salt) per day from all the foods you eat. If you can, cut your sodium intake even more—to no more than 1,500 mg per day, which equals about two-thirds of a teaspoon of salt. Here are some tips on limiting your intake of salt and other forms of sodium:

- Use reduced-sodium or no-salt-added products. Examples are no-salt-added canned vegetables or ready-to-eat cereals that have no added salt or the lowest amount of sodium listed on the Nutrition Facts panel on the food label.
- When you cook, be "spicy" instead of "salty." Flavor foods with herbs, spices, wine, lemon, lime, or vinegar. Be creative!
- Don't bring the salt shaker to the table. Try an herb substitute instead, such as powdered garlic, onion, or thyme.
- Use fresh poultry, fish, and lean meat, rather than canned, smoked, or processed types.
- Cut down on cured foods (such as bacon and ham), foods packed in brine (such as pickles and olives), and condiments (such as mustard, ketchup, barbeque sauce, and monosodium glutamate). You should even limit lower sodium versions of soy sauce and teriyaki sauce.
- Read the Nutrition Facts label on the food package and choose convenience foods that are lower in sodium. These foods include frozen dinners, pizza, breads, packaged mixes, canned soups and broths, and salad dressings.
- Rinse canned foods, such as tuna and canned beans, to remove some of the sodium.

While salt substitutes containing potassium chloride may be useful for some individuals, they can be harmful to people with certain medical conditions. Ask your doctor before trying salt substitutes.

Don't Pass the Salt

What Else Affects Blood Pressure?

A number of foods and other factors have been reported to affect blood pressure. Here are the latest research findings:

Garlic and onions. These foods have not been found to affect blood pressure. But they are tasty, nutritious substitutes for salty seasonings and can be used often.

Caffeine. This may cause blood pressure to rise, but only temporarily. Unless you are sensitive to caffeine, you do not have to limit how much you consume in order to prevent or control high blood pressure.

Stress. Stress, too, can make blood pressure go up for a while, and is popularly thought to contribute to high blood pressure. But the long-term effects of stress are not clear. Furthermore, stress management techniques alone do not seem to prevent high blood pressure. However, stress management approaches may help you control other unhealthy habits, such as overeating or smoking.

High Blood Cholesterol and the TLC Program

TLC is a treatment program that stands for "Therapeutic Lifestyle Changes." This program helps reduce LDL cholesterol via a low-saturated fat, low-*trans* fat, low-cholesterol eating plan. The program also emphasizes regular physical activity and weight control. Adopt the TLC approach and you'll lower your chances of developing heart disease, future heart attacks, and other heart disease complications. (The main difference between the TLC and the DASH eating plans is that the TLC plan puts more emphasis on decreasing saturated fat and *trans* fat to lower blood cholesterol levels.)

Now You're Cooking: Limiting Saturated Fat, *Trans* Fat, and Cholesterol

Planning and preparing nutritious meals may take a little extra effort, but the health benefits are huge. Here are some tips for cutting down on saturated fat, *trans* fat, and dietary cholesterol, which will help lower your LDL cholesterol and reduce your heart disease risk. It will improve heart health for everyone, and may be particularly helpful to those following the TLC eating plan.

Meat, Poultry, and Fish

- Choose fish, poultry, and lean cuts of meat. Trim the fat from meats; remove the skin and fat from chicken. Keep portion sizes moderate.

Taking Charge: An Action Plan for Heart Health

Mineral Medicine:
Another Way To Control Blood Pressure

Certain mineral-rich foods can help keep blood pressure levels healthy. For example, a diet rich in potassium can help to both prevent and control high blood pressure. A potassium-rich diet not only blunts the effects of salt on blood pressure, but may also reduce the risk of developing kidney stones, and possibly decrease bone loss with age. But be sure to get your potassium from food sources, not from supplements. Many fruits and vegetables, some dairy foods, and fish are rich sources of potassium.

Calcium and magnesium are two other minerals that may help to prevent high blood pressure, as well as improve health in other ways. Low-fat or fat-free milk and milk products are rich sources of calcium, while magnesium is found in many whole-grain products; dark green, leafy vegetables; fish; and dry beans.

- Broil, bake, roast, or poach instead of frying. When you do fry, use a nonstick pan and a nonstick cooking spray or a very small amount of oil or margarine.
- Cut down on sausage, bacon, and processed, high-fat cold cuts (which are also high in sodium).

Milk Products and Eggs
- Instead of whole milk or cream, use fat-free or 1-percent milk.
- Use fat-free or low-fat cheeses and yogurt.
- Replace ice cream with sorbet, sherbet, and fat-free or low-fat frozen yogurt. Keep portion sizes moderate.
- Limit the number of egg yolks you eat. Egg whites contain no fat or cholesterol, so you can eat them often. In most recipes, you can substitute two egg whites for one whole egg.
- Use soft margarines (liquid or tub types) that contain little or no *trans* fat. Some brands of soft margarines are high in plant sterols or stanols, which lower LDL cholesterol.

Give Your Heart a Little TLC

If your LDL cholesterol is above your goal level (see page 22), you should start on the TLC eating plan right away. Consuming foods that are high in saturated fat, *trans* fat, and cholesterol contributes to high levels of LDL cholesterol. On the TLC eating plan, you should consume:

- Less than 7 percent of the day's total calories from saturated fat. Lowering saturated fat is the most important dietary change for reducing blood cholesterol.
- Less than 200 milligrams of dietary cholesterol per day.
- Just enough calories to achieve or maintain a healthy weight.

If your blood cholesterol is not lowered enough on the TLC eating plan, your doctor or registered dietitian may advise you to increase the amount of soluble fiber and/or add cholesterol-lowering food products to your diet. These products include margarines that contain "plant sterols" or "plant stanol esters," which are ingredients that lower LDL cholesterol. If your LDL level is still not lowered enough, your doctor may prescribe a cholesterol-lowering drug along with the TLC eating plan. For more information, see NHLBI's Web page, "Live Healthier, Live Longer." (See "To Learn More" on page 88.)

Grains and Grain Products

- Eat foods with lots of fiber and nutrients and make sure that half of your grain products are whole grain. These include whole-grain breads, pasta, and cereals, as well as brown rice. When you check package labels, look for the word "whole" in the ingredients. Make sure that whole grains appear among the first items listed.

Sauces, Soups, and Casseroles

- After making sauces or soups, cool them in the refrigerator and skim the fat from the top. Do the same with canned soups.

- Thicken a low-fat sauce with cornstarch or flour.
- Make main dishes with whole-grain pasta, brown rice, or dry peas and beans. If you add meat, use small pieces for flavoring rather than as the main ingredient.

When You Can't Face Cooking

Check the Nutrition Facts label on food packages to choose frozen dinners and pizzas that are lowest in saturated fat, *trans* fat, and cholesterol. Also watch the calories and sodium content. Make sure the dinners include vegetables, fruits, and whole grains—or add them on the side.

Choose store-bought baked goods that are lowest in saturated fat, cholesterol, *trans* fats, and hydrogenated (hardened) fats. Also, remember that even "no cholesterol" and fat-free baked goods still may be high in calories.

Dining Out for Health

With a little planning and a willingness to speak up you can eat healthfully when you dine out. Here are some tips.

Ask for what you want. Most restaurants will honor your requests. You have nothing to lose by asking!

Order small. To reduce portion size, try ordering appetizers or children's portions as your main meal. Or, take half of your entrée home with you for lunch the next day.

Ask questions. Don't hesitate to ask your server how foods are prepared and whether the restaurant will make substitutions. Ask if they will:

- Serve low-fat or fat-free milk rather than whole milk or cream.
- Tell you the type of cooking oil used. (Preferred types that are lower in saturated fat are canola, safflower, sunflower, corn, and olive oils.)
- Trim the fat off poultry or meat.
- Leave all butter, gravy, and sauces off an entrée or side dish.
- Add no salt during cooking.
- Serve salad dressing on the side.
- Meet special requests if you make them in advance.

Select foods cooked by low-fat methods. Look for terms such as broiled, baked, roasted, poached, or lightly sautéed.

Limit foods high in calories and fats, especially saturated fat and *trans* fat. Watch out for terms such as fried, crispy, creamed, escalloped, hollandaise, bernaise, casserole, and pastry crust.

Make Healthy Choices

- **Breakfast:** Fresh fruit, small glass of citrus juice, low-fat or fat-free milk and yogurt, whole-grain bread products and cereals, omelet made with egg whites or egg substitute.
- **Beverages:** Water with lemon, flavored sparkling water, juice spritzer (half fruit juice and half sparkling water), iced tea, reduced-sodium tomato juice.
- **Breads:** Most yeast breads are low in calories and fat—as long as you limit the butter, margarine, or olive oil. Choose whole-grain breads, which are packed with important nutrients and are full of fiber to make you feel fuller faster. Also, watch the sodium content.
- **Appetizers:** Steamed seafood, fresh fruit, bean soups, salad with reduced-fat dressing.
- **Entrées:** Skinless poultry, fish, shellfish, vegetable dishes, or pasta with red sauce or vegetables. Limit your use of butter, margarine, and salt at the table.
- **Salads:** Fresh lettuce, spinach, and other greens; other fresh vegetables, chickpeas, and kidney beans. Skip high-fat and high-calorie nonvegetable choices such as deli meats, bacon, egg, cheese, and croutons. Choose lower-calorie, reduced-fat, or fat-free dressings, lemon juice, or vinegar.
- **Side Dishes:** Vegetables and grain products, including whole-grain rice or noodles. Ask for salsa or low-fat yogurt instead of sour cream or butter.

■ **Dessert:** Fresh fruit; fat-free frozen yogurt, sherbet, or fruit sorbet (usually fat free, but ask for the calorie content). Try sharing a dessert. If you drink coffee or tea with dessert, ask for low-fat or fat-free milk instead of cream or half-and-half.

Know your foods. Following are some additional tips on shopping, cooking, and eating for heart health:

■ To choose foods wisely, see "How To Use the Nutrition Facts Label on the Food Package" on page 47 and "The Lowdown on Labels."

■ To prepare and eat heart healthy meals, see "Figuring Out Fat" on page 60.

■ For other tips on making good food choices, see "How To Tame a Snack Attack" below and "Vitamins for Heart Health" on page 62.

How To Tame a Snack Attack

Many snacks, including many types of cookies, crackers, and chips, are high in saturated fat, *trans* fat, cholesterol, sodium, and calories. But that doesn't mean you have to cut out all between-meal treats. Keep the foods listed below on hand for snack attacks. But, keep in mind that while these foods may be low in fat, many are not low in calories. So watch how much you eat, especially if you are trying to control your weight.

Here are some healthier, low-fat snacks:

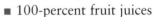

■ 100-percent fruit juices
■ Low-fat or fat-free milk
■ Fat-free frozen yogurt, sherbet, and sorbet
■ Low-fat cookies such as animal crackers, graham crackers, ginger snaps, and fig bars
■ Low-fat crackers such as melba toast, or rice, rye, and soda crackers; look for unsalted or low-sodium types

The Lowdown on Labels

Food labels can help you choose items that are lower in sodium, saturated and total fat, *trans* fat, cholesterol, and calories. When you grocery shop, look for these claims on cans and other packaging—and use this guide to find out what each claim really means.

Sodium Claims	What They Mean
Sodium free or salt free	Less than 5 mg of sodium per serving
Very low sodium	35 mg or less per serving
Low sodium	140 mg or less per serving
Low sodium meal	140 mg or less per 3$\frac{1}{2}$ ounces
Reduced or less sodium	At least 25 percent less per serving than the regular version
Unsalted or no salt added	No salt added during processing

Fat Claims	What They Mean
Fat free	Less than $\frac{1}{2}$ gram of fat per serving
Low saturated fat	1 gram or less of saturated fat per serving
Reduced fat	At least 25 percent less fat per serving than the regular version
Light	50 percent less fat than the regular version

Calorie Claims	What They Mean
Calorie free	Less than 5 calories per serving
Low calorie	40 calories or less per serving
Reduced or less calories	At least 25 percent fewer calories per serving than the regular version
Light or "lite"	Half the fat or one-third of the calories per serving of the regular version

Lowdown on Labels

Figuring Out
Fat

Your personal fat allowance depends on how many calories you consume each day. If you do not have high blood cholesterol or heart disease, the saturated fat in your diet should be less than 10 percent of your daily calories, and total fat should be 20–35 percent of calories. Most fats should come from foods that are high in polyunsaturated fats and monosaturated fats, such as fish, nuts, and vegetable oils.

The table below shows the maximum amount of saturated fat you should eat, depending on how many calories you take in each day. If you have high blood cholesterol or heart disease, the amount of saturated fat will be different. (See "Give Your Heart a Little TLC," on page 55.) Check the Nutrition Facts label on food packages to find out the number of fat grams—both saturated and total—in each serving.

Total Calorie Intake	Limit on Saturated Fat Intake
1,600	18 g or less
2,000*	20 g or less
2,200	24 g or less
2,500*	25 g or less
2,800	31 g or less

Percent daily values on the Nutrition Facts label on the food package are based on a 2,000-calorie diet. Values for 2,000 and 2,500 calories are rounded to the nearest 5 grams to be consistent with the Nutrition Facts label.

Figuring Out Fat

- Fresh or dried fruit, or fruits canned in their own juice
- Vegetable sticks; try a dab of reduced-fat peanut butter on celery sticks
- Air-popped popcorn with no salt or butter; fat-free, low-sodium pretzels

Aim for a Healthy Weight

If you are overweight or obese, taking pounds off can reduce your chances of developing heart disease in several ways. First, losing weight will directly lower your risk. Second, weight loss can help to reduce a number of other risk factors for heart disease, as well as lower your risk for other serious conditions. Weight loss can help control diabetes, as well as reduce high blood pressure and high blood cholesterol. Reaching a healthy weight can also help you to sleep more soundly, experience less pain from arthritis, and have more energy to take part in activities you enjoy.

Remember, if you need to lose weight, even a small weight loss will help lower your risk for heart disease and other serious health conditions. At the very least, you should not gain any additional weight. A recent study found that young adults who maintain their weight over time, even if they are overweight, have lower risk factors for heart disease in middle age than those whose weight increases.

When it comes to weight loss, there are no quick fixes. Successful, lasting weight loss requires a change of lifestyle, not a brief effort to drop pounds quickly. Otherwise, you will probably regain the weight. Aim to lose between 1/2 pound to 2 pounds per week— no more. If you have a lot of weight to lose, ask your doctor, a registered dietitian, or a qualified nutritionist to help you develop a sensible plan for gradual weight loss.

To take off pounds and keep them off, you will need to make changes in both your eating and physical activity habits. Weight control is a question of balance. You take in calories from the foods you eat. You burn off calories during physical activity. Cutting down on calories, especially calories from fat, is key to losing weight. Combining this change in diet with a regular physical activity program, such as walking or swimming, will help you both shed pounds and stay trim for the long term.

Vitamins for Heart Health:
Choose Foods,
Not Supplements

Until recently, it was believed that antioxidant vitamins, particularly vitamin E and beta carotene, might protect against heart disease and stroke, as well as cancer. But new research shows that taking these vitamins in supplement form can be harmful—even deadly.

In the case of vitamin E supplements, a review of 19 studies showed that daily doses of 400 IUs or more may significantly increase the risk of death from all causes. Meanwhile, two major studies showed that supplementation with beta carotene (a substance that is converted to vitamin A in the liver) increases the risks of lung cancer and death in smokers. Other recent studies have shown that there are no benefits to taking either vitamin E or beta carotene supplements to prevent cardiovascular diseases or cancer.

But studies suggest that antioxidants in *foods* do protect heart health. So keep eating plenty of foods that are packed with these vitamins. Foods rich in vitamin E include vegetable oils (especially safflower and sunflower oils), wheat germ, leafy green vegetables, and nuts (almonds and mixed nuts). Foods rich in beta carotene are carrots, yams, peaches, pumpkin, apricots, spinach, and broccoli.

Note: If you are taking vitamin E supplements for protection against medical conditions other than cardiovascular diseases or cancer, talk with your doctor about the risks and benefits of higher dose vitamin E supplements.

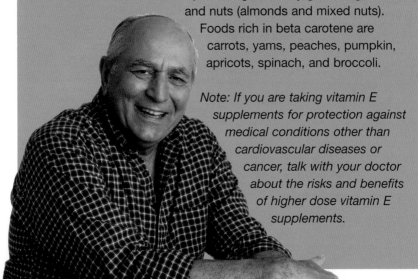

Getting Started

Anyone who has ever tried to lose weight—and keep it off—knows that it can be quite a challenge. Here are some tips to help you succeed:

Eat for health. Choose a wide variety of low-calorie, nutritious foods in moderate amounts. Include vegetables, fruits, whole grains, and low-fat or fat-free milk, as well as fish, lean meat, poultry, or dry beans. Choose foods that are low in fat and added sugars. Choose sensible portion sizes. (See "Portion Distortion" on page 68.)

Watch calories. To lose weight, most overweight people will need to cut 500 to 1,000 calories per day from their current diet.

For tips on choosing low-fat, low-calorie foods, see "The Substitution Solution" on pages 66–67.

Keep milk on the menu. Don't cut out milk products as you try to reduce calories and fat. Milk and milk products are rich in calcium, a nutrient that helps prevent the bone-thinning disease osteoporosis. Instead, choose low-fat or fat-free milk and milk products, which have the same amount of calcium as whole-milk products. Make the switch gradually. If you are used to drinking whole milk, first cut back to 2 percent, then move to 1 percent, and finally to fat-free milk.

Keep moving. Physical activity is key to successful, long-term weight loss. It can help you burn calories, trim extra fat from your waist, and control your appetite. It can also tone your muscles and increase aerobic fitness. To lose weight and to prevent further weight gain, gradually build up to at least 60 minutes of moderate-intensity physical activity on most, and preferably all, days of the week. If you've lost weight, in order to keep it off, you'll need to do even more physical activity—from 60–90 minutes of daily moderate-intensity physical activity. But you don't need to run yourself ragged. A recent study showed that moderate physical activity, such as brisk walking, helps people lose weight as effectively as more vigorous exercise. For more tips, see "Get Moving!" on page 72.

Steer clear of fast food. A single meal from a fast food restaurant may contain as many calories as you need for a whole day! A recent study showed that young adults who eat frequently at fast food restaurants gain more weight and are at higher risk for diabetes in middle age than those who avoid the fast food habit. If you do eat at a fast food restaurant, choose salads and grilled foods, and keep portion sizes small. Ask for salad dressings, mayonnaise, and other high-fat condiments to be served on the side—or not at all.

Know about medicines. If you are very overweight, or if you are overweight and have other weight-related risk factors or diseases, your doctor may advise you to take a medicine to help you take off pounds. You should use a weight-loss drug only after you have tried a low-calorie diet, more moderate-intensity physical activity, and other lifestyle changes for 6 months without successfully losing weight. Because weight-loss medicines have side effects, you should consider all of the risks and benefits before trying one of them. These drugs should be used along with a low-calorie eating plan and regular physical activity, not as a substitute for these lifestyle changes.

Get support. Tell your family and friends about your weight-loss plans and let them know how they can be most helpful to you. Some people also find it useful to join a structured weight-loss program. The most effective groups provide support and advice for permanently changing eating and physical activity habits. (See "How To Choose a Weight-Loss Program" on page 70.)

Lock in your losses. After reaching your weight-loss goal, switch your efforts to keeping the weight off by continuing to eat a nutritious, lower calorie diet and getting regular physical activity. To maintain your weight, you'll need to become even more active than before: Aim for 60 to 90 minutes of physical activity per day. While this may seem like a tall order, remember that you can count the activities that you're already doing. Common daily activities such as climbing stairs, pushing a stroller, unloading groceries, gardening, and brisk walking all count as physical activity. Just be sure you do enough of them!

Seven Secrets of Weight Management

If you have ever tried to take off weight, you know that it's more than a matter of promising yourself that you'll eat less and move more. You also need to mentally prepare yourself for new behaviors. Here are some tips for getting and staying in a healthy weight mindset.

Start small. Many people set unrealistic goals for the amount of weight they want to lose. But you can greatly improve your health by losing just 5 to 10 percent of your starting weight. While you may choose to lose more weight later, keep in mind that this initial goal is both realistic and valuable.

Set smart goals. It's important to set goals that are specific, achievable, and "forgiving" (allow you to be less than perfect). For example, "exercise more" is a fine goal, but it's not very specific. "Walk for 60 minutes every day" is specific and perhaps achievable. But what if you have a bad cold one day, and you awake to a drenching rainstorm on another? "Walk 60 minutes, 5 days each week" is specific, achievable, and forgiving. A great goal!

Build on success. Rather than focusing on one big goal, choose a series of smaller goals that will bring you closer and closer to your larger goal. For example, if one of your big goals is to reduce your daily calories from 2,000 to 1,200, first reduce your calories to 1,700, then move to 1,400, and finally to 1,200. Likewise, with

Thin Quickies:
Are High-Fat, Low-Carb Diets the Way to Go?

The currently popular high-fat, low-carbohydrate diets promise quick, dramatic weight loss. But they're not the route to healthy, long-term weight management. A diet high in fat, especially if it is high in saturated fat, is not good for your heart. These diets are also high in protein and can cause kidney problems and increased bone loss. High-fat, low-carb diets are also low in many essential vitamins, minerals, and fiber.

While some people following this type of a diet lose weight in the short term, much of the weight loss is due to water loss. As with most quick-fix diets, the weight tends to quickly return once you stop dieting. The best course is to steer clear of all fad diets. The healthiest, most effective route to long-term weight loss is a lower fat, lower calorie, well-balanced diet.

The Substitution Solution:
Making the Switch to Low-Calorie Foods

Here are some tasty, low-calorie alternatives to old favorites. Read labels to find out how many calories are in the specific products you buy.

Instead of	Replace With
Milk Products	
Whole milk	Low-fat or fat-free milk
Ice cream	Sorbet, sherbet, fat-free frozen yogurt, or reduced-fat ice cream
Whipping cream	Imitation whipped cream (made with fat-free milk) or low-fat vanilla yogurt
Sour cream	Plain, low-fat yogurt or fat-free sour cream
Cream cheese	Neufchatel cheese, "light" or fat-free cream cheese
Cheese (sandwich types)	Reduced-calorie, low-calorie, or fat-free cheeses
Cereals and Pastas	
Ramen noodles	Brown rice or whole-grain pasta
Pasta with cheese sauce	Whole-grain pasta with red sauce or vegetables
Granola	Bran flakes, crispy rice cereals, cooked grits or oatmeal, reduced-fat granola
Meat, Fish, Poultry	
Cold cuts, hot dogs	Low-fat cold cuts and hot dogs (watch sodium content)
Bacon or sausage	Canadian bacon or lean ham
Regular ground beef	Extra-lean ground beef or ground turkey
Chicken or turkey with skin	White-meat chicken or turkey without skin

Instead of	Replace With
Oil-packed tuna	Water-packed tuna
Beef (chuck, rib, brisket)	Beef (round, loin) with fat trimmed off; if possible, choose select grades
Pork (spareribs, untrimmed loin)	Pork tenderloin (trimmed), lean smoked ham
Whole eggs	Egg whites

Baked Goods

Croissants, brioches, etc.	Hard French rolls or "brown 'n serve" rolls
Donuts, sweet rolls, muffins	English muffins, bagels, reduced-fat or fat-free muffins
Cake (pound, layer)	Cake (angel food, gingerbread)
Cookies	Reduced-fat, low-calorie, or fat-free cookies (graham crackers, ginger snaps, fig bars)

Fats, Oils, Salad Dressings

Regular margarine or butter	Light-spread, reduced-calorie, or diet margarines; look for "*trans* fat-free" soft margarines
Regular mayonnaise	Light or diet mayonnaise
Regular salad dressing	Reduced-calorie or fat-free dressings, lemon juice, vinegars
Butter or margarine on toast	Jelly, jam, or honey on toast
Oils, shortening, or lard	Nonstick cooking spray instead of greasing pans for sautéing

Low-Calorie Foods

Portion Distortion:
How To Choose Sensible Servings

It's very easy to "eat with your eyes" and misjudge what equals a serving—and pile on unwanted pounds. This is especially true when you eat out, because restaurant portion sizes have been steadily expanding. Twenty years ago, the average pasta portion size was 2 cups totaling 280 calories. Today, it's 4 cups totaling 560 calories! To keep your portion sizes sensible:

- When eating out, choose small portion sizes, share an entrée with a friend, or take some of the food home (if you can chill it right away).
- Check the Nutrition Facts label on product packages to learn how much food is considered a serving, as well as how many calories and how much fat are in the food.
- Be especially careful to limit portion sizes of high-calorie foods such as cookies, cakes, other sweets, sodas, french fries, oils, and spreads.

physical activity, first establish a "small" new habit—such as walking 10 minutes a day—and then gradually increase it. Everyone can find time to exercise 10 minutes each day. When you experience success at reaching a small goal, it will motivate you to keep moving toward your larger goals.

Reward yourself! Rewards that you control will encourage you to achieve your goals. For a reward to work well, choose something you really want, don't put off giving it to yourself, and make it dependent on meeting a specific goal. The reward you choose may be something you buy for yourself or an act of self-kindness, such as an afternoon off from your usual responsibilities or an evening spent with a friend. Avoid food as a reward. It usually works better to give yourself frequent, small rewards for reaching short-term goals than bigger rewards that require a long, difficult effort.

BILL KIRWAN

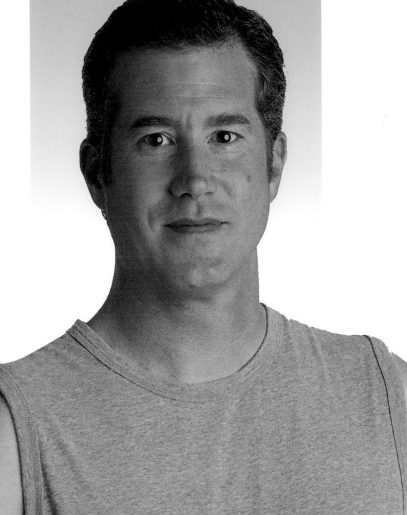

"I realize I'm not as young as I used to be. I began working out doing both weights, and cardio work. Over time the more I exercised, the more I built up, and increased the weights, the more I began to see the benefits. It's a stress reliever. I'm the father of two young boys and they are very active in sports, and now I have the ability to do more of that with them."

Write it down. Regularly record what you do on your weight-loss program, such as your daily calorie intake and amount of physical activity, as well as changes in your weight. (Try to weigh yourself at the same time of day once or twice a week.) Keeping track this way can help you and your health care provider determine what behaviors you may want to improve. Keeping tabs on your progress can also help you stay motivated.

Know your triggers. To lose weight successfully, you'll need to be aware of your personal eating "triggers." These are the situations that usually bring on the urge to overeat. For instance, you may get a case of the munchies while watching TV, when you see treats next to the office coffeepot, or when you're with a friend who loves to snack. To "turn off" the trigger, you'll need to make a change in the tempting situation. Example: If the pile of doughnuts near the coffeepot is hard to resist, leave the scene as soon as you pour yourself a cup of coffee.

The fine art of feeling full. Changing the way you eat can help you eat less without feeling deprived. Eating slowly can help you feel satisfied sooner, and therefore you will avoid second helpings. Eating lots of vegetables and fruits and drinking plenty of noncaloric beverages can also make you feel fuller. Another trick is to use smaller plates and taller, narrower glasses so that moderate portions don't seem skimpy. It can also help to set a regular eating schedule, especially if you tend to skip or delay meals.

How To Choose a Weight-Loss Program

Some people lose weight on their own, while others like the support of a structured program. If you decide to participate in a weight-loss program, here are some questions to ask before you join:

Does the program provide counseling to help you change your eating and activity habits?
The program should teach you how to *permanently* change eating and lifestyle habits, such as lack of physical activity, that have contributed to weight gain. Research shows that people who successfully keep weight off are those who make changes in their overall lifestyles, rather than simply join an exercise program.

Does the staff include qualified health professionals, such as nutritionists, registered dietitians, doctors, nurses, psychologists, and exercise physiologists?

Qualified professionals can help you lose weight safely and success-fully. Before getting started, you'll need to be examined by a doctor if you have any health problems, are currently taking or plan to take any medicine, or plan to lose more than 15 to 20 pounds.

Does the program offer training on how to deal with times when you may feel stressed and slip back into old habits?
The program should provide long-term strategies for preventing and coping with possible weight problems in the future. These strategies might include setting up a support system and a regular physical activity routine.

Do you help make decisions about food choices and weight-loss goals?
In setting weight-loss goals, the program staff should consider your personal food likes and dislikes, as well as your lifestyle. Avoid a "one strategy fits all" program.

Are there fees and costs for additional items, such as dietary supplements?
Before you sign up, find out the total costs of participating in the program. If possible, get the costs in writing.

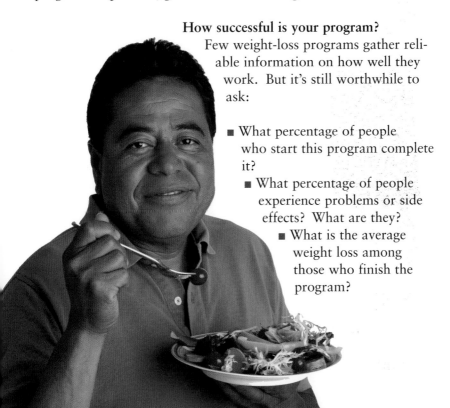

How successful is your program?
Few weight-loss programs gather reli-able information on how well they work. But it's still worthwhile to ask:

- What percentage of people who start this program complete it?
  - What percentage of people experience problems or side effects? What are they?
    - What is the average weight loss among those who finish the program?

Get Moving!

Regular physical activity is a powerful way to reduce your risk of heart disease. Physical activity directly helps prevent heart problems. Staying active also helps prevent and control high blood pressure, keep cholesterol levels healthy, and prevent and control diabetes. Plus, regular physical activity is a great way to help take off extra pounds—and keep them off.

Regular physical activity has a host of other health benefits. It may help prevent cancers of the breast, uterus, and colon. Staying active also strengthens the lungs, tones the muscles, keeps the joints in good condition, improves balance, and may slow bone loss. It also helps many people sleep better, feel less depressed, cope better with stress and anxiety, and generally feel more relaxed and energetic.

You can benefit from physical activity at any age. In fact, staying active can help prevent, delay, or improve many age-related health problems. As you grow older, weight-bearing activities can be particularly helpful for strengthening bones and muscles, improving balance, and lowering the risk for serious falls. Good weight-bearing activities include carrying groceries, walking, jogging, and lifting weights. (Start with 1- to 3-pound hand weights and gradually progress to heavier weights.)

Activities that promote balance and flexibility are also important. Practices such as T'ai Chi and yoga can improve both balance and flexibility and can be done alternately with heart healthy physical activities. Check with your health insurance plan, local recreation center, YWCA or YMCA, or adult education program for low-cost classes in your area.

A Little Activity Goes a Long Way

The good news is that to reap benefits from physical activity, you don't have to run a marathon—or anything close to it. To reduce the risk of disease, you only need to do about 30 minutes of moderate-intensity physical activity on most, and preferably all, days of the week. If you're trying to manage your weight and prevent gradual, unhealthy weight gain, try to boost that level to approximately 60 minutes of moderate- to vigorous-intensity physical activity on most days of the week.

Brisk walking (3 to 4 miles per hour) is an easy way to help keep your heart healthy. One study, for example, showed that regular, brisk walking reduced the risk of heart attack by the same amount as more vigorous exercise, such as jogging. To make physical activity a pleasure rather than a chore, choose activities you enjoy. Ride a bike. Go hiking. Dance. Play ball. Swim. Keep doing physical tasks around the house and yard. Rake leaves. Climb stairs. Mulch your garden. Paint a room.

You can do an activity for 30 minutes at one time, or choose shorter periods of at least 10 minutes each. For example, you could spend 10 minutes walking on your lunch break, another 10 minutes raking leaves in the backyard, and another 10 minutes lifting weights. The important thing is to total about 30 minutes of activity each day. (To avoid weight gain, try to total about 60 minutes per day.)

No Sweat!
Getting regular physical activity can be easy—especially if you take advantage of everyday opportunities to move around. For example:

- Use stairs—both up and down—instead of elevators. Start with one flight of stairs and gradually build up to more.
- Park a few blocks from the office or store and walk the rest of the way. If you take public transportation, get off a stop or two early and walk a few blocks.
- Instead of eating that rich dessert or extra snack, take a brisk stroll around the neighborhood.
- Do housework or yard work at a more vigorous pace.
- When you travel, walk around the train station, bus station, or airport rather than sitting and waiting.
- Keep moving while you watch TV. Lift hand weights, do some gentle yoga stretches, or pedal an exercise bike.
- Spend less time watching TV and using the computer.

Safe Moves

Some people should get medical advice before starting regular physical activity. Check with your doctor if you:

- Are over 50 years old and not used to moderately energetic activity
- Currently have heart trouble or have had a heart attack
- Have a parent or sibling who developed heart disease at an early age
- Have a chronic health problem, such as high blood pressure, diabetes, osteoporosis, or obesity

Once you get started, keep these guidelines in mind:

Go slow. Before each activity session, allow a 5-minute period of slow-to-moderate movement to give your body a chance to limber up and get ready for more exercise. At the end of the warmup period, gradually increase your pace. Toward the end of your activity, take another 5 minutes to cool down with a slower, less energetic pace. It's best to wait until after your activity to do stretching exercises.

Listen to your body. A certain amount of stiffness is normal at first. But if you hurt a joint or pull a muscle, stop the activity for several days to avoid more serious injury. Rest and over-the-counter painkillers can heal most minor muscle and joint problems.

Check the weather report. Dress appropriately for hot, humid days and for cold days. In all weather, drink lots of water before, during, and after physical activity.

Pay attention to warning signals. While physical activity can strengthen your heart, some types of activity may worsen existing heart problems. Warning signals include sudden dizziness, cold sweat, paleness, fainting, or pain or pressure in your upper body just after doing a physical activity. If you notice any of these signs, call your doctor right away.

Use caution. If you're concerned about the safety of your surroundings, pair up with a buddy for outdoor activities. Walk, bike, or jog during daylight hours.

Stay the course. Unless you have to stop your activity for a health reason, stick with it. If you feel like giving up because you think you're not going as fast or as far as you should, set smaller, short-term goals for yourself. If you find yourself becoming bored, try doing an activity with a friend. Or switch to another activity. The tremendous health benefits of regular, moderate-intensity physical activity are well worth the effort.

What's Your Excuse?
We all have reasons to stay inactive. But with a little thought and planning, you can overcome most obstacles to physical activity. For example:

"I don't have time to exercise." While physical activity does take time, remember that you can reduce your heart disease risk by getting just 30 minutes of moderate-intensity physical activity on most days of the week. Plus, you can save time by doubling up on some activities. For example, you can ride an exercise bike or use hand weights while watching TV. Or, you can transform some of your everyday chores—like washing your car or walking the dog—into heart healthy activities by doing them more briskly than usual.

"I don't like to exercise." You may have bad memories of doing situps or running around the track in high school, forcing yourself through every sweating, panting moment. Now we know that you can get plenty of gain without pain. Activities you already do, such as gardening or walking, can improve your health. So just do more of the activities you like. If possible, get your friends or family members involved so that you can support each other.

"I don't have the energy to be more active." Get active first—with brief periods of moderate-intensity physical activity—and watch your energy start to soar. Once you begin regular physical activity, you will almost certainly feel stronger and more vigorous. As you progress, daily tasks will seem easier.

"I want to exercise, but I keep forgetting!" Leave your sneakers near the door to remind yourself to walk, or bring a change of clothes to work and head straight for the gym, yoga class, or walking trail on the way home. Put a note on your calendar to remind yourself to exercise. While you're at it, get in the habit of adding more activity to your daily routine.

Move It and Lose It

Activity	Calories Burned Per Hour*
Walking, 2 mph	240
Walking, 3 mph	320
Walking, 4.5 mph	440
Bicycling, 6 mph	240
Bicycling, 12 mph	410
Tennis, singles	400
Swimming, 25 yards per minute	275
Swimming, 50 yards per minute	500
Hiking	408
Cross-country skiing	700
Jumping rope	750
Jogging, 5.5 mph	740
Jogging, 7 mph	920

For a healthy, 150-pound person. A lighter person burns fewer calories; a heavier person burns more.

You *Can* Stop Smoking

The good news is that quitting smoking immediately reduces your risk of heart disease and other serious disorders, with the benefit increasing over time. Just 1 year after you stop smoking, your heart disease risk will drop by more than half. Within several years, it will approach the heart disease risk of someone who has never smoked. No matter how long you've been smoking, or how much, quitting will lessen your chances of developing heart disease.

Walk Into Health:
A 12-Week Program

Do on most days each week. Your heart will thank you!

Warmup	Activity	Cool Down	Total Time
Week 1 Walk slowly 5 min.	Walk briskly 5 min.	Walk slowly 5 min.	15 min.
Week 2 Walk slowly 5 min.	Walk briskly 7 min.	Walk slowly 5 min.	17 min.
Week 3 Walk slowly 5 min.	Walk briskly 9 min.	Walk slowly 5 min.	19 min.
Week 4 Walk slowly 5 min.	Walk briskly 11 min.	Walk slowly 5 min.	21 min.
Week 5 Walk slowly 5 min.	Walk briskly 13 min.	Walk slowly 5 min.	23 min.
Week 6 Walk slowly 5 min.	Walk briskly 15 min.	Walk slowly 5 min.	25 min.
Week 7 Walk slowly 5 min.	Walk briskly 18 min.	Walk slowly 5 min.	28 min.
Week 8 Walk slowly 5 min.	Walk briskly 20 min.	Walk slowly 5 min.	30 min.
Week 9 Walk slowly 5 min.	Walk briskly 23 min.	Walk slowly 5 min.	33 min.
Week 10 Walk slowly 5 min.	Walk briskly 26 min.	Walk slowly 5 min.	36 min.
Week 11 Walk slowly 5 min.	Walk briskly 28 min.	Walk slowly 5 min.	38 min.
Week 12 Walk slowly 5 min.	Walk briskly 30 min.	Walk slowly 5 min.	40 min.

Walk Into Health

Prepare to Succeed

- **Get motivated.** Take some time to think about all the benefits of being "smoke free." Besides the health benefits of quitting, what else do you have to gain? Money saved from not buying cigarettes? Loved ones no longer exposed to secondhand smoke? A better appearance? No more standing outside in the cold or rain for a smoke? Write down all of the reasons you want to stop smoking.
- **Sign on the dotted line.** Write a brief contract that states your intention to stop smoking, your quitting date, and some ways you plan to reward yourself for becoming an exsmoker. Have someone sign it with you.
- **Lineup support.** Ask the person who cosigns your contract—or another friend or relative—to give you special support in your efforts to quit. Plan to get in touch with your support person regularly to share your progress and to get encouragement. If possible, quit with a friend or family member.

Breaking the Habit

- **Know yourself.** To quit successfully, you need to know your personal smoking "triggers." These are the situations and feelings that typically bring on the urge to light up. Some common triggers are drinking coffee, having an alcoholic drink, talking on the phone, watching someone else smoke, and experiencing stress. Make a list of your own personal triggers. Especially during the first weeks after quitting, try to avoid as many triggers as you can.
- **Find new habits.** Replace your "triggers" with new activities that you don't associate with smoking. For example, if you've always had a cigarette with a cup of coffee, switch to tea for a while. If stress is a trigger for you, try a relaxation exercise such as deep breathing to calm yourself. (Take a slow, deep breath, count to five, and release it. Repeat 10 times.)
- **Keep busy.** Get involved in activities that require you to use your hands, such as needlework, art projects, jigsaw puzzles, or fix-up projects around your house or apartment. When you feel the urge to put something in your mouth, try some vegetable sticks, apple slices, or sugarless gum. Some people find it helpful to inhale on a straw or chew on a toothpick until the urge passes.
- **Keep moving.** Walk, garden, bike, or do some yoga stretches. Physical activity will make you feel better and will help prevent weight gain.

ALAN LETOW

"My father died of heart problems. I'm on medication for my high blood pressure. I'm trying to learn from my family history by focusing on maintaining my quality of life. I don't want to get old. I want to be able to do all the things I have been doing all my life. I am a little kid at heart."

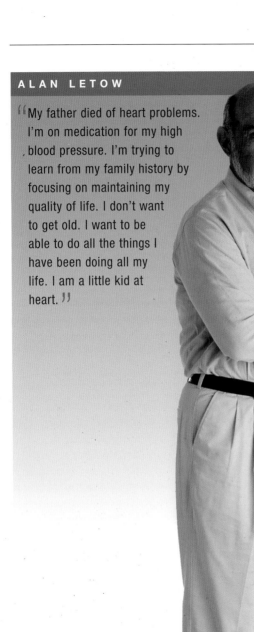

- **Know what to expect.** During the first few weeks after quitting, you may experience temporary withdrawal symptoms such as headaches, irritability, tiredness, and trouble concentrating. While these feelings are not pleasant, it may help to know that they are signs that your body is recovering from smoking. Most symptoms end within 2 to 4 weeks.
- **Ask for help.** A number of free or low-cost programs are available to help people stop smoking. They include programs offered by local chapters of the American Lung Association and the American Cancer Society. Other low-cost programs can be found through hospitals, health maintenance organizations, workplaces, and community groups.
- **Give yourself a break.** Get plenty of rest, drink lots of water, and eat three healthy meals each day. If you are not as productive or cheerful as usual during the first weeks after quitting, be gentle with yourself. Give yourself a chance to adjust to your new smoke-free lifestyle. Congratulate yourself for making a major, positive change in your life.

More Help for Quitting

As you prepare to quit smoking, consider using a medicine that can help you stay off cigarettes. Some of these medications contain very small amounts of nicotine, which can help lessen the urge to smoke. They include nicotine gum (available over-the counter), the nicotine patch (available over the counter and by prescription), a nicotine inhaler (by prescription only), and a nicotine nasal spray (by prescription only). Another quitting aid is Bupropion SR, a medicine that contains no nicotine but reduces the craving for cigarettes. It is available only by prescription. While all of these medications can help people stop smoking, they are not safe for everyone. Talk with your doctor about whether you should try any of these aids.

Help for Quitting

If You "Slip"
A slip means that you've had a small setback and smoked a cigarette after your quit date. Most smokers slip three to five times before they quit for good. To get right back on the nonsmoking track:

- **Don't be discouraged.** Having a cigarette doesn't mean you can't quit smoking. A slip happens to many people who successfully quit. Keep thinking of yourself as a nonsmoker. (You are one.)
- **Learn from experience.** What was the "trigger" that made you light up? Were you driving home from work, enjoying a glass of wine at a party, feeling angry with your boss? Think back on the day's events until you remember what the trigger was.
- **Take charge.** Write a list of things you will do the next time you face that particular trigger situation—and other tempting situations as well. Sign a new contract with your support person to show yourself how determined you are to kick the habit. You're on your way.

A **Weighty** Concern

Many people fear that if they stop smoking, they will gain unwanted weight. But most exsmokers gain less than 10 pounds. Weight gain may be partly due to changes in the way the body uses calories after smoking stops. Some people also may gain weight because they substitute high-calorie foods for cigarettes. Choosing more low-calorie foods and getting more physical activity can reduce the amount of weight you gain.

If you do put on some weight, you can work on losing it after you have become comfortable as a nonsmoker. When you consider the serious health risks of smoking, the possibility of gaining a few pounds is no reason to continue.

A Weighty Concern

Aspirin: Take With **Caution**

This well-known "wonder drug" is an antiplatelet medicine that can help to lower the risk of a heart attack or stroke for those who have already had one. Aspirin also can help to keep arteries open in those who have had a heart bypass or other artery-opening procedure, such as angioplasty. In addition, aspirin is given to people who arrive at the hospital with a suspected heart attack or stroke.

It's important to know that aspirin has not been approved by the U.S. Food and Drug Administration for the prevention of heart attacks in those who have never had a heart attack or stroke.

However, a recent, large study has found that among healthy women, taking low-dose aspirin every other day may help to prevent a first stroke, and among women over the age of 65, may also help prevent a first heart attack. If you are considering taking aspirin for this purpose, keep in mind that it is a powerful drug with many side effects, and can mix dangerously with other drugs. Take daily aspirin to prevent heart attack only with your doctor's specific advice and guidance. If aspirin is a good choice for you, be sure to take the dose recommended by your doctor.

If you're thinking about using aspirin to either prevent or treat a heart problem, talk with your doctor first. Only a doctor who knows your medical history and current health condition can judge whether the benefits would outweigh the risks. If aspirin is a good choice for you, be sure to take the dose recommended by your doctor.

If your doctor does advise you to take aspirin, be sure to continue practicing the "Big Four" heart healthy habits—eating nutritiously, getting regular physical activity, maintaining a healthy weight, and avoiding smoking. While aspirin can be a useful treatment for some people, it is not a substitute for a healthy lifestyle.

Heart Health Is a Family Affair

When it comes to heart health, what's good for you is good for your whole family—including its youngest members. We now know that two-thirds of teenagers have at least one risk factor for heart disease, from overweight and "couch potato-itis" to unhealthy blood pressure and cholesterol levels. Even more disturbing, about one million U.S. teenagers have metabolic syndrome, which is a cluster of risk factors that greatly increases the risk of a later heart attack. We owe it to our children and grandchildren to help them develop heart healthy habits—and the earlier the better. Here are some ways to begin:

Set a good example. Adults have a big influence on children's and teens' behavior—even though kids may not want to admit it. If you follow a healthy lifestyle, the younger members of your family will be more likely to do the same. Let them see you eating nutritious snacks and enjoying outdoor activities, and invite them to join in. If you smoke, stop—and tell your kids and grandkids why you're quitting.

What's cookin'? Fully 80 percent of children eat fewer than five servings of fruits and vegetables per day. What to do? Practice "stealth cooking"—creating healthy meals for kids that will still make their mouths water. You can chop veggies into small pieces and add them to favorite recipes, such as pizza or spaghetti sauce. If your kids love tacos, try replacing taco shells with crunchy lettuce leaves, and pile on some extra chopped tomato. Use whole-wheat or bran breads to add fiber to sandwiches. For dessert, skip the ice cream and offer fresh fruit, fig bars, ginger snaps, graham crackers, or frozen fat-free dairy desserts.

Raise "kitchen kids." Most children enjoy cooking when it's presented as an easy, fun activity. Show young kids how to clean fruits and veggies and combine them into colorful salads. Let them make "fruit-salad faces" out of sliced apples, bananas, and raisins. When they're old enough, teach children to use the stove, oven, microwave, and toaster safely. Show teens how to make simple, healthy dishes, such as whole-grain pasta with vegetables and broiled chicken or fish. Encourage them to be creative with herbs and spices. Children who have basic kitchen skills appreciate food more and are more likely to try new dishes.

Get them moving. The latest "Dietary Guidelines for Americans" recommend that children and teenagers be physically active for at least 60 minutes per day. Yet, in a world chock full of video games, TV shows, and computer offerings, few young people are as active as they should be. To encourage children to get off the couch, find out what kinds of physical activities they do enjoy and make it easy for them to participate. If the kids in your family like to ride bikes, plan a Sunday outing on your local trail. Walk, cycle, or jog with them to places close by. Use your backyard or local park to toss a Frisbee around or to play a game of basketball, badminton, or volleyball. Make an effort to gear activities to children's ages. Younger kids, up to age 10, tend to have quick bursts of energy sandwiched between longer periods of rest, while older children usually have more endurance. Play down the competition, play up the fun, and pretty soon, your kids may start asking *you* to shoot some hoops. Better get in shape!

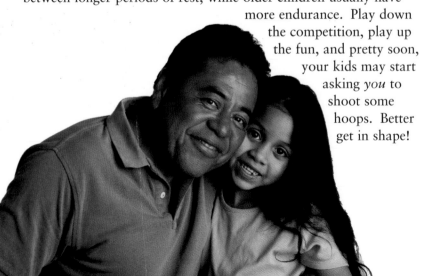

A Change of Heart

Taking care of your heart is one of the most important things you can do for your health and well-being. But, because heart health involves changing daily habits, it can require some real effort. To make the process easier, try tackling only one habit at a time. For example, if you smoke cigarettes and also eat a diet high in saturated fats, work first on kicking the smoking habit. Then, once you've become comfortable as a nonsmoker, begin to skim the fat from your diet.

Remember, nobody's perfect. Nobody always eats the ideal diet or gets just the right amount of physical activity. The important thing is to follow a sensible, realistic plan that will gradually lessen your chances of developing heart disease.

So keep at it. Work with your doctor. Ask family members and friends for support. If you slip, try again. Be good to your heart, and it will reward you many times over—with a better chance for a longer, more vigorous life.

How To Estimate Your Risk
Estimate of 10-Year Risk for Men

Age	Points
20–34	-9
35–39	-4
40–44	0
45–49	3
50–54	6
55–59	8
60–64	10
65–69	11
70–74	12
75–79	13

	Points				
Total Cholesterol	Age 20–39	Age 40–49	Age 50–59	Age 60–69	Age 70–79
<160	0	0	0	0	0
160–199	4	3	2	1	0
200–239	7	5	3	1	0
240–279	9	6	4	2	1
≥280	11	8	5	3	1

	Points				
	Age 20–39	Age 40–49	Age 50–59	Age 60–69	Age 70–79
Nonsmoker	0	0	0	0	0
Smoker	8	5	3	1	1

HDL (mg/dL)	Points
≥60	-1
50–59	0
40–49	1
<40	2

Systolic BP (mmHg)	If Untreated	If Treated
<120	0	0
120–129	0	1
130–139	1	2
140–159	1	2
≥160	2	3

Point Total	10-Year Risk %
<0	<1
0	1
1	1
2	1
3	1
4	1
5	2
6	2
7	3
8	4
9	5
10	6
11	8
12	10
13	12
14	16
15	20
16	25
≥17	≥30

10-Year risk_____%

How To Estimate Your Risk
Estimate of 10-Year Risk for Women

Age	Points
20–34	-7
35–39	-3
40–44	0
45–49	3
50–54	6
55–59	8
60–64	10
65–69	12
70–74	14
75–79	16

Total Cholesterol	Points				
	Age 20–39	Age 40–49	Age 50–59	Age 60–69	Age 70–79
<160	0	0	0	0	0
160–199	4	3	2	1	1
200–239	8	6	4	2	1
240–279	11	8	5	3	2
≥280	13	10	7	4	2

	Points				
	Age 20–39	Age 40–49	Age 50–59	Age 60–69	Age 70–79
Nonsmoker	0	0	0	0	0
Smoker	9	7	4	2	1

HDL (mg/dL)	Points
≥60	-1
50–59	0
40–49	1
<40	2

Systolic BP (mmHg)	If Untreated	If Treated
<120	0	0
120–129	1	3
130–139	2	4
140–159	3	5
≥160	4	6

Point Total	10-Year Risk %
<9	<1
9	1
10	1
11	1
12	1
13	2
14	2
15	3
16	4
17	5
18	6
19	8
20	11
21	14
22	17
23	22
24	27
≥25	≥30

10-Year risk_____%

To Learn More

The National Heart, Lung, and Blood Institute provides information on the prevention and treatment of heart disease and offers publications on heart health and heart disease.

NHLBI Health Information Center
P.O. Box 30105
Bethesda, MD 20824-0105
Phone: 301–592–8573
TTY: 240–629–3255
Fax: 301–592–8563

NHLBI Heart Health Information Line
1–800–575–WELL
Provides toll-free recorded messages.

Also, check out these heart health Web sites and Web pages:

NHLBI Web site: www.nhlbi.nih.gov

Diseases and Conditions A–Z Index:
http://www.nhlbi.nih.gov/health/dci/index.html

The Heart Truth: A National Awareness Campaign for Women About Heart Disease: www.hearttruth.gov

Your Guide to Lowering High Blood Pressure: www.nhlbi.nih.gov/hbp/index.html

Live Healthier, Live Longer (on lowering elevated blood cholesterol): www.nhlbi.nih.gov/chd

High Blood Cholesterol: What You Need To Know:
www.nhlbi.nih.gov/health/public/heart/chol/hbc_what.htm

Aim for a Healthy Weight:
www.nhlbi.nih.gov/health/public/heart/obesity/lose_wt/index.htm

Act in Time to Heart Attack Signs: www.nhlbi.nih.gov/actintime/index.htm

Heart Healthy Recipes:
www.nhlbi.nih.gov/health/public/heart/other/syah/index.htm
http://www.nhlbi.nih.gov/health/public/heart/other/ktb_recipebk/

Smoking Cessation: For information from the National Cancer Institute on quitting smoking, call 1–800–QUITNOW
(1–800–784–8669) or go to http://www.smokefree.gov/

For still more information on heart health, see Medline Plus:
http://medlineplus.gov/